Voss Health™

Building the Systems that Create Health

The Willpower Lie

Why Obesity Isn't a Character Problem—and How We Can Build a World That Makes Health Easier

Copyright and Medical Disclaimer

The Willpower Lie: Why Obesity Isn't a Character Problem—and How We Can Build a World That Makes Health Easier

Published by Medical Specialists Associates, PC.

This book is intended for general educational and informational purposes only. It is not intended to provide individualized medical advice, diagnosis, or treatment, and it should not be used as a substitute for professional medical care. Readers should consult a qualified physician or other licensed healthcare professional before making decisions about medications, surgery, nutrition, weight management, exercise, or any other health-related intervention.

Obesity, metabolic disease, diabetes, sleep apnea, cardiovascular disease, liver disease, eating disorders, and other medical conditions require individualized evaluation and care. Nothing in this book establishes a physician-patient relationship between the author and the reader. Any discussion of medical treatment, medication, surgery, nutrition, or lifestyle intervention is presented in general terms and may not apply to every individual.

Readers should not start, stop, or change any medication, supplement, diet, exercise plan, or medical treatment based solely on information in this book. Any urgent or emergency medical concern should be addressed immediately by contacting emergency services or seeking care from an appropriate healthcare professional.

Although the author has made reasonable efforts to present accurate and current information, medical knowledge, clinical guidelines, medications, and treatment recommendations may change over time. The author and publisher disclaim any liability for any loss, injury, or damage allegedly arising from the use or application of information contained in this book.

Any examples, patient-like scenarios, or clinical illustrations in this book are intended to clarify concepts and should not be interpreted as specific medical advice for any individual reader.

First edition.
ISBN: 979-8-90434-011-7
Printed in the United States of America

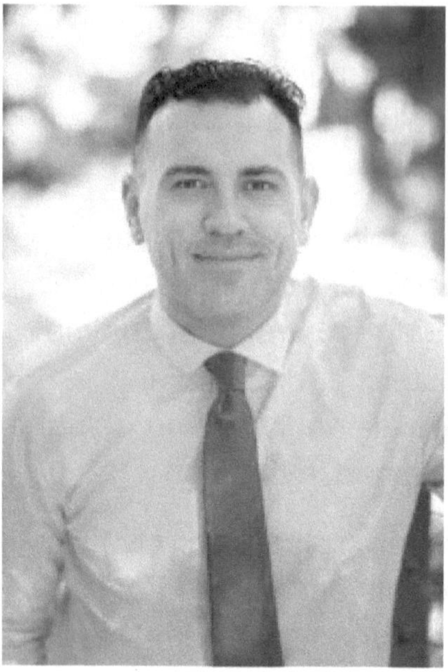

Christopher Voss, MD, MBA, MS, MLS, FCCP, is a physician, physician executive, author, and healthcare entrepreneur whose work spans obesity medicine, lifestyle medicine, critical care, pain medicine, addiction medicine, clinical informatics, and healthcare leadership. He is board-certified in Obesity Medicine and Lifestyle Medicine, as well as in Anesthesiology, Critical Care Medicine, Pain Medicine, Neurocritical Care, Addiction Medicine, Clinical Informatics, and Healthcare Administration, Leadership, and Management. He also holds board certifications in perioperative transesophageal echocardiography and critical care echocardiography and is a Fellow of the American College of Chest Physicians.

Dr. Voss earned his medical degree from Tulane University School of Medicine and completed a two-year research fellowship at the National Cancer Institute, part of the National Institutes of Health. He trained in surgery at Stanford University School of Medicine, in anesthesiology at the University of

California, San Francisco and Emory University School of Medicine, and in Critical Care Medicine and Pain Medicine at Brigham and Women's Hospital, Harvard Medical School. He also earned an MBA and a Graduate Certificate in Health Sector Management from Duke University, completed healthcare leadership training through the California Healthcare Foundation–UCSF program, earned a Master's degree in Maharishi Ayurvedic and Integrative Medicine, completed graduate training in health information technology at Columbia University, and earned a Master's degree in Legal Studies with a concentration in Business Law from Washington University in St. Louis.

He is president of Medical Specialists Associates, PC, a multispecialty, multistate medical group with a significant focus on telemedicine, and has held clinical and leadership roles across anesthesiology, intensive care, pain medicine, and addiction medicine.

Dr. Voss is the author of *Counterfeit Fulfillment: How Conditioning Fuels Addiction—and How Integration Restores Freedom*, *The Care Divide: Two Lives, Two Systems, and the Case for Universal Healthcare*, and *The System Doesn't Sell Health: Why We Pay More, Get Less, and Struggle to Stay Well*.

In this book, Dr. Voss brings together clinical medicine, obesity care, systems leadership, healthcare economics, and a commitment to human dignity to argue for a more humane and effective approach to metabolic health. His work emphasizes that obesity should be treated with scientific seriousness and compassion, while also challenging the upstream environments, incentives, and food systems that make health harder to sustain. The central argument of this book is that obesity medicine must move beyond downstream rescue and help reshape the conditions that produce disease in the first place.

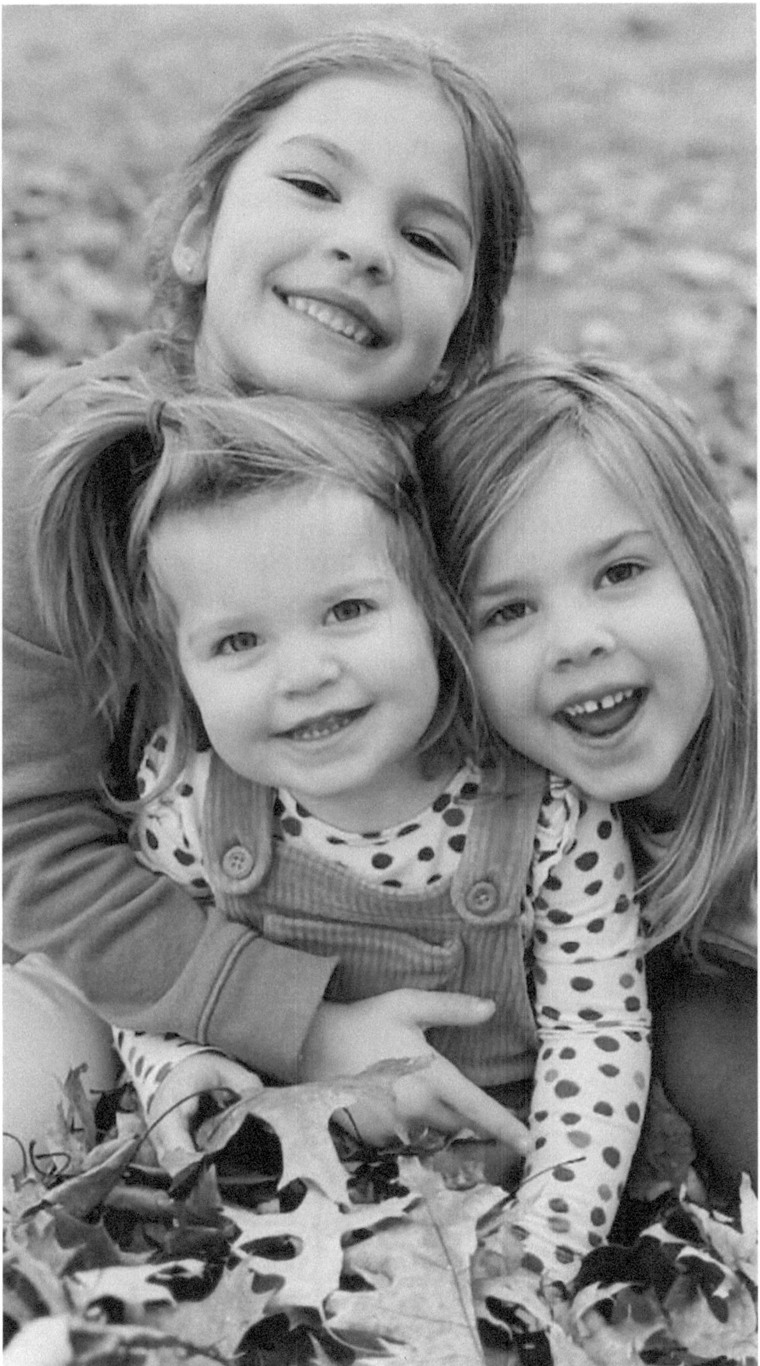

Dedication

To my daughters,

I wrote this book with your future in mind.

My hope is that you inherit a world that tells the truth with compassion, a world that understands health without shame, and a world that does not ask individuals to carry alone the weight of systems built around exhaustion, convenience, and disease.

I want you to grow up in a culture that protects dignity, supports real nourishment, honors rest, and makes the healthier path easier for more people to walk. I want you to know that medicine should not only rescue people after harm is done, but should also help build the conditions that make health more possible in the first place.

This book is dedicated to you because you remind me why that work matters.

May the world you inherit be wiser, kinder, and healthier than the one we have too often accepted.

Table of Contents

Prologue: The Missing Fourth Line

It is early evening, and the day has already made many decisions for the person who is about to eat.

Work ran late. Traffic was heavy. The children are hungry. The kitchen is still dark. A grocery store offers a long wall of brightly packaged convenience, a hot bar built for speed, and a produce section that asks for more money, more time, more planning, and more energy than the moment seems to have available. Across town, an airport traveler walks through a food court where the fastest options are also the easiest to overeat. In a school hallway, in an office break room, at a gas station, in a hospital vending area, the same pattern repeats. Cheap, easy, engineered calories are ready. Better options, when they exist, usually ask more of an already tired life.

That is not a trivial detail. It is the beginning of the story.

For years, the national conversation about obesity has been dominated by a narrow idea: that body weight is mostly a matter of personal discipline, and that rising obesity must therefore reflect some broad decline in personal responsibility. That story is emotionally satisfying to people who do not look closely. It is also incomplete in a way that has harmed millions of people.

It has harmed them medically, because it has pushed the country toward shallow explanations for a serious disease. It has harmed them morally, because it has told people to feel blame where they often should have been given understanding. And it has harmed them strategically, because when a nation misdiagnoses a problem, it builds the wrong solutions.

This book begins from a different premise. Modern obesity is not primarily a failure of individual character. It is the predictable result of an environment that has become increasingly good at driving overconsumption and increasingly bad at supporting metabolic health. Ultra-processed food, low-cost calories, chronic stress, insufficient sleep, time scarcity, larger portions, frequent eating cues, and schedules that wear people down before dinner all matter. They do not remove human agency. They do explain why agency becomes harder to sustain at scale.

I write this as a physician who treats obesity and metabolic disease, and as a physician leader who has spent enough time inside healthcare systems to see a troubling pattern. We have become more sophisticated at recognizing downstream disease. We have become more capable of paying for downstream treatment. But we are still too willing to leave the upstream conditions intact and then act surprised by the results. We should not be.

There is a simple way to organize the science at the center of this book.

Quantity in calories influences body weight.
Quality of macronutrient balance, especially protein adequacy, influences body composition.
Quality of nutrient density influences health.
Environment determines how hard or easy it is to live out the first three.

That is the framework. It is simple on purpose. But simple is not the same as simplistic.

The first line matters because energy still matters. However much nutrition discourse changes, body weight does not float free from calorie balance. But the first line is not enough. A person can lose weight in ways that leave them weaker, hungrier, and less healthy than they should be. That is why the second line matters. What your body is made of is not the same thing as what your body weighs. Body composition means the balance of body fat, muscle, and other lean tissue. In real life, that distinction changes everything. The goal is not simply to become lighter. The goal is to reduce excess body fat while preserving strength, function, and health.

The third line matters because a body is not fed by calories alone. Food carries information as well as energy. A diet can be low in calories yet poor in protein, fiber, vitamins, minerals, and overall quality. It can move the scale while leaving the biology undernourished. Weight is not the whole story. A number on the scale cannot tell you whether the food supporting that number is building health or quietly eroding it.

And then there is the fourth line.

The fourth line is the part our culture keeps leaving out. It is the missing line in countless conversations about food, discipline, and health. It is the difference between nutrition as a tidy theory and nutrition as human life.

Environment determines how hard or easy it is to live out the first three.

That line does not cancel the other three. It makes them real.

People do not live inside theory. They live inside prices, schedules, fatigue, advertising, portion sizes, school food, workplace food, commute times, family stress, neighborhood access, sleep debt, and the options that happen to be within reach when the day is almost over. A person can know what to do and still be surrounded by conditions that make doing it predictably harder. Knowledge matters. Biology matters. Choice matters. But environment determines the level of friction.

That truth helps explain one of the most important facts in modern health: obesity did not become widespread because millions of people all suffered the same sudden collapse in virtue. Widespread disease usually points to widespread exposure. When a condition becomes common enough, a culture starts mistaking prevalence for normality. But common is not the same as healthy. Familiar is not the same as harmless.

This point requires care, because obesity is one of the most stigmatized conditions in public life and in medicine. Many people living with obesity have been lectured, dismissed, blamed, or reduced to a stereotype. Some have been made to feel that their body size reflects laziness, ignorance, weak character, or some private moral failure. Some have heard that message from strangers. Some from family. Some from clinicians. Some have delivered it to themselves for years.

If that is part of your story, this book is not written to shame you. It is not written to mock you, flatten you, or place you on trial. It is written to make the problem clearer, and clarity is one form of respect.

But respect must not become denial. This is another place where the national conversation often fails.

A humane society should reject weight stigma. It should also reject the idea that obesity is merely cosmetic, or that disease becomes less real because it has become common. People deserve dignity at every body size. They also deserve honesty about health risk, metabolic strain, and the real burden that excess body fat—especially when it is dysregulated or stored in higher-risk patterns—can place on the body over time. Truth and compassion are not opposites. In good medicine, they belong together.

This book will return often to another distinction that gets lost in everyday conversation: weight is not the same as health. Nor is weight the same as body composition. Those differences matter because people can chase smaller numbers on a scale and miss the more important target. Losing fat while preserving muscle is not the same as simply weighing less. A stronger body with better metabolic health is not the same as a smaller body achieved at any cost. In an age obsessed with visible change, we need a more serious definition of improvement.

That is also why this book is not hostile to treatment. It is not an anti-medication book. It is not an anti-surgery book. Modern obesity medicine has tools that can be life-changing. For many people, evidence-based medications can reduce appetite, improve metabolic health, and create breathing room after years of struggle. For selected patients, metabolic and bariatric surgery can be transformative. These treatments deserve respect. They should not be caricatured, dismissed, or morally downgraded.

But they should also not become the whole story.

Rescue matters. Rescue is honorable. Rescue relieves suffering. But rescue is not the same as redesign.

If we rely only on downstream treatment, we accept a future in which the environment keeps generating disease while medicine becomes increasingly busy managing the consequences. That is not balance. That is surrender dressed up as sophistication. A nation cannot fully medicate its way out of a food environment that is pushing millions of people in the wrong direction. It cannot operate its way out of time poverty, chronic exhaustion, and a daily landscape dominated by cheap, engineered calories. The better answer is not less treatment. It is a wider lens.

That wider lens changes more than the obesity conversation. It changes what we ask of healthcare, of employers, of schools, of insurers, of business leaders, and of physicians.

For too long, medicine has often been asked to stand at the downstream end of the problem, documenting blood sugar after it rises, prescribing blood pressure medications after it climbs, managing fatty liver after it appears, treating sleep apnea after it develops, and addressing obesity after years of exposure have already done their work. Some of that will always be necessary. Caring for the patient in front of us is a moral duty. But it is not our only duty.

If the healthcare system can justify paying for expensive treatment after disease is established, it should at least be willing to take seriously the conditions that make disease more likely in the first place. Healthy food access should not be treated as a lifestyle luxury floating outside real medicine. It should increasingly be understood as a medically meaningful intervention. The same profession that prescribes powerful drugs should be willing to ask harder questions about why vegetables, fruit, quality protein, and healthier staple foods remain more difficult to access than the cheap calories that reliably worsen metabolic health.

This is not an anti-business argument. Markets matter. Work matters. Productivity matters. Innovation matters. The problem is not that economic systems exist. The problem is that incentives decide what those systems make easy, profitable, and widely available. When the strongest incentives reward shelf life, speed, convenience, hyper-palatability, and low cost per calorie more than nutrient density and long-term health, the outcomes should not surprise us. The engine is real. The target matters.

By the end of this book, I want the reader to see obesity with a steadier, wider, and more humane frame. I want you to understand why obesity became normal in the culture without becoming normal health. I want you to see why body weight alone is too crude a measure of progress. I want you to understand why protein, muscle, sleep, stress, and time scarcity matter more than the public conversation usually admits. I want you to see where medications and surgery fit, and why they matter, while also seeing why they cannot be the whole national answer. I want you to see why physicians should move some of their influence further upstream. And I want you to consider the possibility that business incentives, insurance design, and public policy can be redirected toward health rather than disease.

Above all, I want this book to replace a punishing story with a truer one.

The punishing story says that people failed first, and the system merely stood by. The truer story is that the system changed first, and then human biology did what human biology does when it is repeatedly exposed to easy energy, low-friction overconsumption, poor recovery, and chronic strain. That does not erase personal responsibility. It places responsibility where it has always belonged: on individuals, yes, but also on the environments, institutions, and incentives that shape what is possible for millions of people at once.

We cannot solve a systems problem by pretending it is only a character problem. We cannot care well for patients while refusing to examine the world that keeps making care necessary. And we cannot keep confusing what is common with what is healthy.

To move forward, we have to retire one of the most stubborn myths in modern health.

The country did not suddenly lose willpower.

Chapter One: The Country Did Not Suddenly Lose Willpower

That sentence at the end of the prologue is not a slogan. It is a diagnostic rule.

If one person struggles with weight, you can tell an individual story. If millions of people begin struggling in the same rough era, across different regions, households, and backgrounds, you need a population story. Broad disease patterns rarely begin with a broad collapse in virtue. They begin when the conditions of ordinary life change.

The moral-failure story has lasted so long because it is simple, emotionally neat, and flattering to people who are not living under the same pressure. It turns a national pattern into a private verdict. It lets the observer feel disciplined, the system feel innocent, and the solution sound easy. Try harder. Eat less. Show some restraint.

But a tidy explanation is not the same as a true one.

Some people who have not struggled much with weight are sincere when they believe discipline is the whole answer. What they often do not see is how much their own biology and environment may have quietly helped them. Appetite differs. Satiety differs. Household routines differ. Income, sleep, commute length, stress burden, family structure, and food access differ. When restraint costs one person less, it is easy for that person to mistake lower friction for higher virtue.

The personal-failure story is also convenient for institutions. If obesity is mostly a matter of character, then the larger design of daily life can remain largely unexamined. Food companies can keep selling what sells. Retail environments can keep placing the easiest calories in the easiest reach. Schools, employers, insurers, and policymakers can talk about wellness while leaving most defaults untouched. The burden stays private. The system keeps its distance.

That is not how serious health thinking is supposed to work.

In medicine, when something becomes common, we are supposed to ask what changed in the exposure, not merely what changed in the person. If a neighborhood begins having more asthma, we look at air, housing, smoke, mold, and pollution. If injuries rise on a stretch of road, we inspect the road. If an infection spreads, we look for vectors, contact, and conditions of transmission. We do not begin by assuming that millions of people all suffered the same synchronized moral lapse. Obesity deserves that same level of seriousness.

That is especially true because human biology did not rewrite itself in a generation. Our genes did not suddenly become unrecognizable. The basic machinery of hunger, reward, fullness, energy storage, and stress response is ancient. What changed much faster were the surroundings: the food supply, the pace of life, the availability of calories, the disappearance of natural stopping points, the amount of sleep people get, the pressure under which they make decisions, and the degree to which the day now places food in front of them long before real hunger has spoken.

Different people carry different vulnerabilities, of course. Genetics matter. Early-life exposure matters. Hormones matter. Medications matter. Trauma matters. Sleep matters. Two people can live in the same broad environment and not respond in the same way. But vulnerability is not the same thing as cause. Susceptibility tells us who may struggle more. It does not erase the fact that the conditions around them changed.

It is also important to say what this argument is not. It is not the claim that human choice is meaningless. Choice matters. Responsibility matters. Agency matters. But choice never occurs in a vacuum. It occurs inside a structure. The structure can support judgment or grind it down. It can create barriers against excess or remove them one by one. It can make a healthier pattern more reachable, or it can keep offering cheap, fast, engineered calories to people who are tired, rushed, stressed, under-slept, and trying to get through the day.

That difference matters because self-regulation is not some mystical force floating above biology. It is influenced by hunger, sleep, stress, routine, mood, time, money, and what is within reach. A rested person with a plan, a stocked kitchen, and time to prepare food is not living the same nutritional life as a person who is running late, commuting home, juggling children, answering messages, and standing in front of a wall of convenience food. To pretend those are the same test of character is not honesty. It is blindness.

In many parts of modern life, people are asked to be nutritionally exceptional just to avoid predictable metabolic harm. That is one reason the willpower story rings so hollow to anyone who has looked closely. The environment has become so saturated with low-friction calories that moderation often requires unusual vigilance. Not occasional vigilance. Daily vigilance. Repeated vigilance. Vigilance in grocery stores, in office break rooms, at school events, in airports, at gas stations, during long drives, after long shifts, and in the tired hour when dinner still has to happen.

This is not because people became uniquely weak. It is because the modern environment became uniquely persistent.

Food is more available, more portable, more shelf-stable, more heavily marketed, and more ready to eat than at any earlier point in history. Eating has drifted away from clearly bounded meals toward a culture of constant opportunity. The body is asked to decide again and again and again. Should I have this now? Should I finish this? Should I buy this for later? Should I say no for the fifth time today? Even before we talk about calories, that repetition matters.

It matters even more when the available foods are built not just to nourish, but to sell, store, travel, and tempt. Many of these products solve real problems. They are cheap. They last. They are fast. They fit busy lives. None of that is trivial. Convenience is not a fake need. For millions of households, it is one of the central realities of modern life.

But the same features that make foods easy to distribute and easy to buy can also make them easy to overconsume. When calories arrive quickly, when textures invite fast eating, when portions are large, when drinks deliver energy without much fullness, when snacks become background rather than events, the body can take in a great deal before the mind fully registers what happened. The body is not indifferent to speed, reward, and repeated exposure.

Much of eating is not a grand decision at all. It is repetition. What is stocked gets eaten. What is visible gets remembered. What is convenient gets used. What is normal gets copied. A great deal of daily behavior runs on default rather than on deliberate philosophy. That is true in finance, in transportation, in sleep, and certainly in food. When defaults are built around convenience-first calories, the results should not surprise us.

The point is not that every processed food is poison or that every convenience food is a trap. The point is that a food environment can be built in ways that steadily favor excess over regulation. A culture can create meals with fewer natural brakes. It can reward speed over satiety, shelf life over freshness, and low cost per calorie over nutrient quality. Then it can act shocked when waistlines, blood sugar, fatty liver, blood pressure, and sleep apnea begin to rise together.

Add to that the quiet force of time poverty.

Many households are not making food decisions from a place of calm abundance. They are making them in between obligations. They are making them when a child needs to be picked up, when a shift runs late, when money is tight, when the refrigerator is thin, when energy is low, when the commute has already taken too much, and when the thought of washing, chopping, cooking, and cleaning feels larger than the remaining bandwidth of the evening. Under those conditions, convenience stops being a luxury and becomes a lifeline. The market knows that. So does biology.

Then there is sleep. Then stress. Then the mental load of a life that rarely settles. An exhausted brain does not think about food the way a restored brain does. A stressed body does not bargain with appetite the way a recovered body does. That is not laziness. That is physiology meeting modern life. We will come back to those forces later in the book, because they deserve their own careful attention. For now, it is enough to see that the obesity story is not only about what is on the plate. It is also about the conditions under which the plate is chosen.

Once you see the problem that way, the idea of mass moral collapse begins to look less like insight and more like evasion.

The country did not wake up one morning and decide to become less disciplined. Parents did not suddenly stop caring about their children's health. Patients did not collectively agree to enjoy struggle. What changed was the exposure. The current grew stronger. The calories became easier. The stopping points weakened. The recovery needed for restraint became harder to protect. The pressure became ordinary.

That last point matters.

Pressure became ordinary.

And when pressure becomes ordinary, it disappears from view.

This is one reason widespread obesity becomes so easy to misunderstand. Ubiquity changes perception. Once a condition becomes common enough, the eye adjusts. Large portions start to look normal. Constant snacking starts to look normal. Sugary drinks start to look normal. Meals eaten in cars start to look normal. Short sleep starts to look normal. Quiet exhaustion starts to look normal. A day structured around convenience starts to look not just common, but inevitable.

Culture adapts quickly to what it sees every day, even when the body is paying a price for the adaptation.

That is dangerous, because common is not the same as healthy. A disease-producing environment does not become benign just because it becomes familiar. If anything, familiarity can make it harder to challenge. People begin to believe that this is simply how modern life works, that higher average body weight, worsening blood sugar, declining fitness, increasing liver fat, and chronic low energy are just what happens now. The background starts to feel like destiny.

But it is not destiny. It is design, exposure, and repeated default.

Here, too, we need care. To say that obesity has become common is not to say that every person with a higher body weight has the same level of risk, the same body composition, or the same health profile. It is not to say that a number on a scale tells the whole story. It does not. Some people at lower weights are metabolically unwell. Some people at higher weights function far better than they are often assumed to. Weight is a clue, not a full biography.

That distinction matters because one of the failures of the public conversation has been its crudity. It has often treated body size as if it were the whole story of health, and then treated that crude story as a moral one. Neither move serves patients well. We will need a more precise conversation about body composition, fat distribution, muscle, function, and metabolic risk than the culture usually offers. But precision should sharpen the conversation, not blur it. It should move us beyond caricature, not into denial.

That is why this chapter has to hold two truths at once.

The first is that the moral-failure story is false.

The second is that false blame is not the only danger. False reassurance is a danger too.

Some people hear a systems explanation and worry that it excuses everything. It does not. It explains more, which is different. Explanation is not surrender. It is how serious people locate leverage. If a bridge is failing because its supports have been compromised, we do not answer with better speeches about careful walking. We inspect the structure. We repair the load-bearing parts. People still have to cross wisely. But wisdom alone is not a substitute for sound design.

The same is true here. A systems view does not erase the role of personal decisions. It puts those decisions where they belong: inside a larger reality of prices, stress, availability, habit, marketing, sleep, recovery, and biological susceptibility. It refuses the fantasy that discipline alone can reliably outmaneuver an environment built to keep pushing in the opposite direction. And it refuses the cruelty of telling people that their repeated struggle proves they did not care enough.

In clinic, that cruelty has a cost.

Shame does not improve metabolic health. It more often drives silence, avoidance, and self-blame. It makes people delay care. It pushes conversations underground. It can turn every failed attempt into evidence against a person's worth instead of evidence that the strategy, the support, or the environment was not strong enough to sustain them. A patient who has struggled many times does not usually need more accusation. More often, that patient needs a truer map.

A truer map begins with compassion, but it cannot end there. Compassion without clarity becomes sentimentality. Clarity without compassion becomes contempt. Neither helps. People deserve dignity at every size. They also deserve honesty about what obesity can do to the body over time and why treatment, when needed, is medically serious rather than cosmetic. This is not a choice between kindness and truth. In good medicine, respect and truth travel together.

That has implications beyond the clinic. Once obesity is understood as a systems-shaped disease rather than a simple referendum on character, the field of responsibility widens. Food manufacturers matter. Retail environments matter. School food matters. Neighborhood access matters. Insurance design matters. Public policy matters. So do the rhythms of work, sleep, transportation, and family life. None of those forces removes human agency. All of them shape how much friction agency must overcome.

This is not an anti-business argument. It is an incentive argument. Markets are powerful. They scale what is rewarded. If reward flows most easily toward foods that are cheap, durable, convenient, intensely appealing, and profitable at scale, those foods will dominate the landscape. That is not a moral mystery. It is how systems behave. The problem is not that economic engines exist. The problem is what we have asked those engines to produce.

It is also not an anti-patient argument. Patients are not the problem that has to be corrected. They are the people living inside the problem. That distinction matters more than it may seem. When the story changes, the posture changes. The conversation becomes less accusatory and more useful. Instead of asking, “Why can’t people control themselves?” we begin asking better questions. What are they up against every day? Which parts of the environment keep defeating their best intentions? What would make healthier eating easier to sustain, not just easier to recommend? Where has medicine accepted downstream rescue while leaving upstream damage mostly untouched?

Those questions are more demanding than the old ones. They ask more of healthcare leaders, policymakers, educators, employers, insurers, food companies, and physicians. They ask more of me as well. It is always easier to lecture a person than to confront a system. But easy explanations are part of how this problem became so entrenched. Serious disease deserves more serious thinking.

The country did not suddenly lose willpower.

It became more exposed.

It became more saturated with calories that are easy to access, easy to eat quickly, and hard to stop.

It became more tired.

It became more rushed.

It became more accustomed to a food landscape that asks very little before giving a great deal of energy back.

And then, too often, it was told to interpret the result as a private moral weakness.

We can do better than that.

We can tell the truth about obesity without humiliating people.

We can respect treatment without pretending treatment alone will solve the deeper problem.

We can admit that body weight matters without confusing weight with the whole story of health.

And we can stop asking individuals to carry all the moral weight for a system that has been quietly redesigning daily life around overexposure, under-recovery, and cheap convenience.

If the moral story is too small, we need a better frame. We need a model that ordinary people can remember, one that is simple enough to teach without becoming simplistic. We need a way to separate weight from body composition, diet quality from mere calorie count, and personal effort from the environment that either supports that effort or steadily wears it down.

That is where we turn next.

Chapter Two: The Simple Science of Food

If the last chapter cleared away a false story, this chapter offers a better map.

At some point in almost every obesity clinic, the conversation narrows to a tired, honest question.

What am I actually supposed to believe about food?

The question usually comes after years of mixed messages. Count calories. Stop counting calories. Cut fat. Cut carbs. Eat more often. Stop snacking. Fast longer. Never skip breakfast. Skip breakfast every day. Eat clean. Be flexible. Trust your body. Ignore your cravings.

By the time people ask the question, they are usually not asking for novelty. They are asking for relief from confusion.

They want a framework they can remember.

That desire is more reasonable than it may sound. Nutrition has been turned into a cultural argument when, for most people, it first needs to become a practical one. A person trying to lose excess body fat, preserve muscle, lower blood sugar, feed a family, stay within a budget, and still have enough energy to get through the week does not need another ideology. That person needs a model that is simple enough to teach and nuanced enough to respect reality.

One reason food advice becomes so noisy is that people keep trying to answer different questions with one sentence.

Why did body weight go up?

What kind of weight is being gained or lost?

Is this pattern of eating actually supporting health?

And can a real human being live this way in real life?

Those are not the same question. So they should not be forced into the same answer.

The model at the center of this book is meant to keep those questions in order:

Quantity in calories influences body weight.
Quality of macronutrient balance, especially protein adequacy, influences body composition.
Quality of nutrient density influences health.
Environment determines how hard or easy it is to live out the first three.

That is the model.

It is simple on purpose.

But simple is not the same as simplistic.

Each line does a different job. The first helps explain body weight. The second helps explain what that weight is made of. The third helps explain whether the body is being well supported. The fourth explains whether the first three can actually be sustained outside a textbook.

Body weight is one question.

Body composition is another.

Health is another.

Adherence is another.

When those questions are collapsed into one, nutrition gets confusing. When they are separated and then placed back together, it becomes more truthful and more useful.

The first line is the one people know best, even if they are tired of hearing about it.

Quantity in calories influences body weight.

A calorie is a unit of energy. It is not a moral point. It is not a measure of virtue. It does not tell you whether a food is nourishing, but it does tell you that energy is entering the system.

Over time, body weight is influenced by the relationship between the energy coming in and the energy being used. However fashionable it becomes to deny that, the body does not stop obeying physiology.

That truth is sometimes delivered in a way that makes people feel blamed, and that is part of why the conversation has become so charged. Many readers have heard some version of the same small, dismissive message: calories matter, therefore your struggle must be simple. But the second half of that sentence does not follow from the first.

Calories matter. That is true.

It does not mean weight regulation is emotionally easy, biologically identical from person to person, or socially uncomplicated. It does not mean appetite is the same in every body. It does not mean medications, sleep, stress, hormones, genetics, trauma, or the food environment are irrelevant. It does not mean a person can effortlessly regulate intake while living inside constant exposure, chronic fatigue, and low-friction convenience food.

The fact that calories matter is not a verdict against anyone. It is simply part of the physiology.

That distinction matters because many people swing between two bad conversations. One conversation says calories are all that matter, as if hunger, fullness, food quality, and sustainability barely exist. The other says calories do not matter at all, as if energy balance can be talked out of the body by sheer theory.

Neither view is serious enough.

A more honest sentence would sound like this: calories matter, but they do not act alone. They interact with appetite, satiety, food quality, sleep, stress, routine, and the environment in which a person is trying to live.

That is why some people find calorie awareness useful and others find it exhausting. A tool is not the same thing as the physiology underneath it. A person may choose to track intake closely, loosely, or not at all. Different people can use different methods. But whatever method is used, body weight does not become exempt from energy balance.

Still, the first line is only the first line.

A scale can tell you that mass changed. It cannot tell you whether the change made you stronger or weaker, better nourished or less nourished, more functional or less functional. It cannot tell you whether the weight that changed was mostly fat, muscle, water, or some combination of all three.

That is why the second line matters so much.

Quality of macronutrient balance, especially protein adequacy, influences body composition.

Macronutrients are the major components of food that provide energy and structure: protein, carbohydrate, and fat. All three matter. All three can have a place in a healthy pattern of eating. But they do not do the same work in the body, and that difference becomes especially important in obesity treatment.

Protein deserves special attention here because it helps do something patients are too rarely taught to protect: lean mass.

Lean mass includes muscle and other non-fat tissue. In everyday language, this is part of what gives the body strength, structure, and function. Muscle matters for movement, metabolism, resilience, and independence. It matters when a person gets up from a chair, climbs stairs, carries groceries, recovers from illness, or simply wants to feel capable in daily life.

That is why body composition matters.

Body composition means what the body is made of. Not just how much it weighs, but how much of that weight is body fat and how much is lean tissue.

This is one of the most important distinctions in the entire book, and one of the most neglected in the public conversation. Two people can each lose twenty pounds and not have the same result at all. One may lose a meaningful amount of excess body fat while preserving strength and function. The other may become lighter while also becoming weaker, hungrier, and less physically capable than before.

The scale records both stories as success.

The body does not.

A smaller body is not always a healthier body if the path to getting smaller strips away too much of what should have been protected.

That is one reason protein adequacy matters so much during weight loss. When calories come down, the body does not always take energy only from the exact tissue we would prefer. If protein is too low, if food quality is poor, if strength is not being maintained, or if weight loss is pursued in a careless way, valuable lean tissue can be lost along with body fat.

Patients deserve a better target than “weigh less.”

The better target is to reduce excess body fat while protecting as much strength, function, and muscle as possible.

Protein can help with that in more than one way. It provides building material for the body. It can also improve fullness, which makes many eating patterns easier to sustain. A meal built around adequate protein often lands differently than one built mostly around refined starch, added sugar, or low-satiety convenience calories. The person may feel fuller for longer. The afternoon may go differently. The number of repeat decisions required before dinner may go down.

That matters.

Because the hard part of nutrition is often not knowing what is healthy. The hard part is living in a way that does not leave a person hungry, depleted, and vulnerable to the next easy calorie.

None of this means carbohydrate is the villain, or fat is the villain, or that every person must eat the same way. Nutrition becomes foolish when it turns into a courtroom and one nutrient is dragged to the defendant's table every few years.

Carbohydrates can range from highly refined, easy-to-overeat products to fiber-rich foods that support health and satiety. Fats are energy-dense and important, and different fats behave differently in real diets. Protein is not magic, but it is often underprotected in weight-loss efforts that focus only on eating less.

The point is not to join another nutrition tribe. The point is to understand that what fills the plate influences what is preserved, what is lost, how full a person feels, and how well the body functions during the process.

That is why "weight loss" can be too crude a phrase when used carelessly.

If the weight being lost includes too much muscle, the apparent victory may come with a hidden cost.

If the strategy leaves a person constantly hungry, it may not last.

If the number on the scale falls while strength, energy, and food quality fall with it, that is not the full kind of progress people were promised.

The second line is there to protect readers from that confusion.

Then comes the third line.

Quality of nutrient density influences health.

If calories tell us how much energy a food provides, nutrient density helps tell us what useful nutrition comes with that energy.

A food pattern can be high in calories and low in useful nourishment. It can also be modest in calories and still leave the body poorly supported if protein, fiber, vitamins, minerals, and overall quality are consistently weak. This is one of the strange features of the modern food environment: a body can be heavily exposed to calories and still be poorly fed in ways that matter.

A person can be overfed in energy and undernourished in quality at the same time.

That is not a contradiction. It is one of the defining problems of modern eating.

Food does more than move the scale. It helps shape blood sugar, fullness, digestion, recovery, blood pressure, blood lipids, liver health, and longer-term disease burden. It affects how steady a person feels, how often hunger returns, and whether the body is receiving what it needs to function well over time.

That is why weight and health should never be treated as interchangeable.

A lower number on the scale cannot tell you whether the diet behind that number is truly supporting health. A person can lose weight on a poor-quality diet. That does not make it a good long-term diet. It simply means the first line moved while the third line may have been neglected.

This is where nutrient density becomes so important. Foods that bring protein, fiber, vitamins, minerals, and other helpful components along with their calories generally support health differently than foods that deliver energy with relatively little else.

That does not require nutritional perfection. It does not require moral purity. It does not require pretending that every meal will be beautifully composed and home-cooked.

It simply means the body is affected not only by how much food it receives, but by what kind of food keeps arriving.

The body notices.

A meal pattern built mostly from minimally processed foods, adequate protein, fiber-rich plant foods, and better-quality staples usually supports health differently than one built mostly from ultra-processed convenience calories. The difference shows up not just in long-term disease risk, but often in fullness, energy, cravings, and day-to-day function.

This matters because many people have been taught to reduce nutrition to one narrow question: did the scale go down?

But health asks more from food than that.

Did the food help preserve muscle?

Did it support blood sugar and fullness?

Did it provide useful nourishment?

Did it leave the person more capable of sustaining a healthier pattern tomorrow?

Those questions are not extras. They are part of the real job.

That is also why the phrase "eat less" is too incomplete to be very useful on its own.

At best, it captures part of the first line.

At worst, it leaves out everything that determines whether the first line can be achieved without damaging the second, neglecting the third, and collapsing under the fourth.

Eat less what?

Eat less in what structure?

Eat less while getting enough protein?

Eat less while preserving strength?

Eat less while staying full enough that the evening does not become the hardest part of the day?

Eat less while living on a tight budget, after a long commute, with children to feed, under stress, and with a refrigerator that may or may not be fully stocked?

A slogan is not a strategy.

"Eat less" is directionally true in the same way "be financially responsible" is directionally true. It points in a general direction. It does not tell a person how to structure the days, handle the pressures, protect the essentials, or survive repeated exposure.

This is one reason so many people feel they have failed nutrition advice when, in reality, the advice failed to match the size of the problem.

If a person tries to lose weight by sheer restriction, without enough protein, without attention to food quality, without regard for hunger, without a plan for the workweek, the result may be brief success followed by exhaustion, overeating, or rebound. Then the person is tempted to interpret the outcome as personal weakness.

But often the deeper truth is simpler than that.

The map was too small.

A patient does not need to hear only that calories matter. A patient needs to know how to lower excess calories without abandoning muscle, without hollowing out diet quality, and without pretending that real life will stop being real life.

That is what the fourth line is for.

Environment determines how hard or easy it is to live out the first three.

The first three lines explain what tends to happen inside the body.

The fourth explains what tends to happen inside a life.

This is the line that turns nutrition from a narrow personal lesson into a broader human one. It is also the line that keeps the model honest.

Because a nutrition plan that sounds excellent in theory may fail every weekday at 6:30 p.m.

A healthy eating pattern that assumes endless time, stable money, easy access, predictable schedules, cooking confidence, good sleep, low stress, and a supportive food environment is not really a population model. It is a private fantasy for the unusually resourced.

Real people live inside prices, commute times, family demands, work schedules, neighborhood options, school schedules, grocery access, marketing, fatigue, cultural norms, and the level of food preparation their day can actually tolerate.

That is not a side issue.

That is the setting in which all nutrition guidance either survives or dies.

The fourth line does not cancel personal agency. It explains friction. It helps us understand why the same nutritional truth can be easy for one person to live and brutally difficult for another. It explains why a rested person with a stocked kitchen and a quiet evening is taking a different test than a tired person standing under fluorescent lights at a gas station or driving home late past a row of fast-food windows.

In that sense, the fourth line is where physiology becomes policy.

It is the bridge between the clinic and the culture.

A model that leaves out environment may describe metabolism. It does not fully describe modern life.

And modern life matters. Because when the easiest available foods are cheap, heavily marketed, low in protein, low in fiber, easy to eat quickly, and hard to stop eating, then all three of the earlier lines can drift in the wrong direction at once. Calories rise more easily. Body composition is harder to protect. Diet quality falls. Health suffers. The person is then told to solve the whole problem with more discipline.

That is not a complete understanding of nutrition. It is nutrition with the hardest part removed.

This is why the fourth line belongs in the model from the beginning rather than as an afterthought. A person does not merely need to know what is biologically true. A person needs some reasonable chance of being able to live by it.

That is the difference between advice and design.

It is also the difference between blaming and leading.

Once the model is clear, many apparent contradictions in nutrition stop being contradictions at all. A person can lose weight without improving diet quality very much. Another person can improve food quality and fullness before the scale changes dramatically. Another may increase protein, start preserving more muscle, and feel better before major weight loss occurs. Another may know exactly what to do but live in conditions that make doing it repeatedly difficult.

The model helps make sense of those different stories.

It tells us that body weight matters, but it is not the whole story.

It tells us that what the body is made of matters, not just what the body weighs.

It tells us that nourishment matters beyond calorie count alone.

And it tells us that adherence is not a character test floating outside the world.

That last point is one of the most important in the whole book.

People do not live inside theory.

They live inside systems.

That is why the four-part model is not just a nutrition lesson. It is a way of seeing the larger problem clearly.

Quantity in calories influences body weight.

Quality of macronutrient balance, especially protein adequacy, influences body composition.

Quality of nutrient density influences health.

Environment determines how hard or easy it is to live out the first three.

People need a model they can remember because the culture keeps giving them slogans that are too small.

This model is meant to be larger than a slogan and simpler than a textbook.

It is meant to be usable.

And once you hold it in your mind, the modern food environment starts to look different. It stops looking like a random collection of personal temptations and starts looking more like a system that can disrupt all four lines at once. It can make calories easier to exceed, protein and muscle harder to protect, nutrient density easier to neglect, and adherence harder to sustain.

That is where we turn next.

The modern food supply does not merely offer food. It often makes overconsumption easier than regulation, convenience easier than nourishment, and repeated exposure stronger than intention. To understand obesity clearly, we have to look closely at that design.

Chapter Three: Engineered to Overeat

No one wakes up in the morning and decides, with full ceremony, that today will be a day of overeating.

The pattern is usually quieter than that.

A sweetened coffee on the commute because breakfast did not happen. A few handfuls from a box in the break room because lunch is late. A snack in the car because traffic is crawling and dinner is still far away. Something crunchy after dinner because the day has been long and the bag is open. By the time many people begin wondering why their intake feels so hard to control, the answer is already in front of them. Much of modern eating is no longer organized around true hunger, clear meals, and obvious stopping points. It is organized around exposure.

That is what this chapter is about.

In ordinary conversation, the phrase processed food often starts the wrong argument. It can sound like a purity test, a moral drama, or a demand that busy families somehow live as if modern life never happened. That is not the argument here. This chapter is not a plea for perfection, and it is not an attack on any household that relies on packaged or ready-to-eat foods. Millions of people do, often because they have to. Convenience is not a fake need. It is one of the central facts of modern life.

But we still need to tell the truth about what kind of convenience our systems have built.

Many foods in the modern marketplace are not merely prepared. They are optimized. They are designed to last longer, travel farther, cost less per serving, require little preparation, deliver a strong sensory reward, and be easy to eat quickly and often. Those goals make commercial sense. In many cases they also make daily life easier. But when those same goals are applied again and again across a national food supply, they can create something larger than convenience. They can create a system in which overconsumption becomes easier than moderation.

That distinction matters. It shifts the conversation away from the tired question, "Why can't people just choose better?" and toward a more serious one: What exactly have we placed in front of people, all day, every day, in what form, at what speed, and with how little friction?

Food engineering is not a conspiracy theory. It is product design.

Companies make decisions about ingredients, texture, shelf life, packaging, portion size, flavor intensity, portability, and price. They decide whether a product will be soft or crunchy, sippable or chewable, subtle or highly flavored, individually wrapped or sold in a large container, marketed as a meal or carried around as a snack. They decide how long it can sit on a shelf, how consistently it performs, how much preparation it requires, and how easily a customer can say yes again tomorrow. Those are ordinary commercial decisions.

They are not metabolically neutral decisions.

A product can be excellent at surviving a shelf and poor at satisfying a body.

In fairness, most product design meetings do not begin with the question, "How can we worsen metabolic health?" They begin with questions that sound commercially practical and morally unremarkable. How do we make this stable? How do we make it affordable? How do we make it taste good, travel well, hold up in heat, appeal to children, fit a cupholder, survive shipping, or earn repeat sales? The metabolic consequence appears downstream. But once a predictable downstream effect becomes visible across a population, the system cannot keep pretending that design and health have nothing to do with each other.

A food product does not have to be harmful by intent to be mismatched with human appetite. It only has to be very easy to eat, very rewarding, and very available. If enough calories can be delivered with enough speed and enough pleasure, repeated often enough, the biology tends to do the rest.

This is one reason the phrase ultra-processed food matters, even if it is imperfect and sometimes overused. Not all processing is the problem. Freezing vegetables is processing. Canning beans is processing. Yogurt is processed. Cheese is processed. Whole-grain bread, frozen fruit, and many practical staples that help real families eat better are processed in some way. Human beings have always processed food.

The more important question is what kind of processing took place, for what purpose, and with what effect on eating behavior.

Ordinary cooking usually begins with recognizable foods and changes them into a meal. An egg is cooked. Potatoes are roasted. Oats are turned into breakfast. Chicken is seasoned and baked. Beans are simmered. A salad is assembled. Even when those meals are enjoyable and energy-dense, they usually retain some features that make eating more self-limiting. They require preparation. They are eaten at a table more often than out of a package. They often involve chewing, serving, pausing, and stopping. They tend to have clearer beginnings and endings.

By contrast, many ultra-processed products are industrial formulations built largely from refined starches, sugars, oils, isolates, flavor systems, and additives that help with texture, consistency, color, shelf life, and repeated appeal. They are often designed to be ready to eat, hard to spoil, easy to transport, and easy to consume before fullness has much time to organize a response. That does not mean every such product is equally harmful, or that all minimally processed foods are automatically superior in every context. It means the structure of the food has changed in ways that often change what happens next.

What happens next is not just nourishment.

What happens next is eating behavior.

This is where many public conversations go shallow. They focus almost entirely on the nutrition label, as if food were only a delivery vehicle for numbers. Calories matter. Protein matters. Fiber matters. But food is also physical. It has texture, volume, speed, crunch, softness, aroma, temperature, sweetness, saltiness, richness, and what might be called ease of continuation. Some foods ask a body to work through the experience. Others slip past almost before the body has had time to register what arrived.

That difference matters more than most people realize.

A body does not feel calories directly. It responds to a cluster of signals. How much volume came in. How much chewing happened. How fast the food arrived. How much protein and fiber were present. Whether the calories came as liquid, puree, crunch, or intact whole food. Whether eating happened as a meal or as repeated small episodes that barely felt like eating at all. Fullness is real, but it is not instantaneous. Satiety is part biology, part timing, part food structure, and part circumstance.

When calories arrive in forms that are softer, faster, more refined, more energy-dense, and easier to eat with little interruption, intake can rise almost without announcing itself.

That is one reason the phrase hyper-palatable has entered the discussion. It is a technical phrase for a simple idea. Some foods are not just tasty. They are unusually easy to keep eating. The combination of fat, sugar, refined starch, salt, flavoring, and engineered texture can create a level of reward that exceeds what most ordinary home cooking is trying to do. To be clear, delicious food is not the enemy. Pleasure is part of eating and part of life. The problem is not that food tastes good. The problem is when a large share of the food environment is built to make stopping unusually difficult.

There is a difference between a meal being enjoyable and a product being optimized for continued intake.

People can also overeat home cooking, restaurant food, holiday food, and minimally processed food. Industrial formulation does not hold a monopoly on excess. The more serious claim is different: the modern food system has scaled excess into an everyday, portable, repeatable form. It has made highly rewarding eating available not only on special occasions, but in the car, at the desk, between errands, after school, during meetings, in the checkout lane, and late at night when judgment is tired and convenience feels earned.

I am also careful not to turn every strong preference into addiction language. Not every appealing food is an addiction, and not every repeat purchase deserves a clinical label. But the brain does learn from repeated reward. Cues matter. Smells matter. Colors, wrappers, jingles, and routines matter. A food system that repeatedly pairs convenience with strong sensory reward should not be surprised when those products become habitual.

That line is easy to miss because modern food is so normalized. A person tears open a bag, opens a pouch, twists a cap, unwraps a bar, or drives away with a cup in the console, and the act feels ordinary. But ordinariness can hide design. The food may have been built to hit quickly, built to taste consistent every time, built to stay shelf-stable for months, built to be eaten while distracted, and built to ask almost nothing before the next bite.

This is not a small point. It helps explain why the obesity conversation has to go beyond food ignorance.

Many people already know what healthier eating generally looks like. They know vegetables matter. They know soda is not the same as water. They know protein matters more than the culture often implies. They know a fast-food meal eaten in the car most nights is probably not a strong long-term plan. The problem is not that nobody understands anything. The problem is that understanding must now compete with a food system that keeps making the easier option highly rewarding, highly visible, and highly repeatable.

That competition is not fair.

Even in carefully controlled research settings, when people are given diets made from more heavily processed foods versus minimally processed foods, they often eat more on the ultra-processed pattern and gain weight more easily, even when the meals appear similar on paper in several major nutrient categories. One of the lessons from that work is that food does not act only through labels and intentions. The form of the food matters. The speed of eating matters. The structure of the diet matters. What looks similar in theory may behave very differently in a real body.

That helps explain something clinicians see all the time. A person may tell you, quite sincerely, "I don't feel like I eat that much." Often that statement is not denial at all. It is a clue. The person may not be experiencing their intake as a series of large, dramatic meals. The intake may be arriving through quiet accumulation: liquid calories that did not feel like food, handfuls that did not feel like a meal, fast eating that outran awareness, convenient snacks that were present long before hunger was fully formed, and portions that no longer look especially large because the culture has resized normal.

This is why passive overconsumption matters so much.

Passive overconsumption is not a binge, not a spectacle, and not necessarily a loss of control in the dramatic sense people imagine. It is intake that drifts upward because the environment makes calories easy to consume without requiring much intention. A person does not sit down and declare a plan to overeat. The day simply keeps offering foods that are dense, rewarding, accessible, and easy to continue. The body receives the energy whether or not the moment felt significant enough to count.

A muffin on the run. A large drink that can be finished before real fullness says much of anything. Chips from a communal bowl. A "snack" package that contains dessert-level calories but is marketed as casual fuel. Candy at a checkout lane. A protein bar that is helpful in some contexts but becomes one more background calorie when the day is already crowded with them. A sweetened coffee that lands more like a small meal while still feeling, psychologically, like a beverage.

None of these examples is a moral scandal on its own.

That is exactly why they matter.

The body does not only respond to what we meant to eat. It responds to what we kept putting in front of it.

The obesity epidemic was not built mainly from dramatic episodes. It was built, in large part, from ordinary ones. From the quiet surplus. From the repeated convenience. From food forms that made calories easy to take in before satiety fully arrived. From days in which eating became less like a bounded act and more like a lightly managed background process.

Some of this is about energy density. Certain foods pack a large amount of energy into a relatively small volume, which means a person can eat a lot of calories before the stomach and brain have much reason to call time out. But energy density is only part of the story. Speed matters too. A food that is easy to chew, easy to swallow, easy to drink, and easy to keep reaching for does not give fullness the same chance to keep pace that a slower, more intact, more protein- and fiber-supportive meal often does.

The body's brakes can work.

But they can be outrun.

This is one reason liquid calories deserve special attention in any honest conversation about overeating. A sugary drink, a sweetened coffee beverage, a shake built more like dessert than nourishment, or a large juice can deliver substantial energy with very little chewing and often surprisingly little fullness in return. Again, the point is not that every such drink is forbidden. The point is that a modern environment filled with high-calorie beverages changes how much energy can enter a day almost invisibly. A person can consume a meaningful amount before dinner and still feel as if dinner is the main event.

Solid foods can be built in similar ways. A potato asks one kind of interaction. Potato chips ask another. Oatmeal with fruit and nuts asks one kind of pace. A pastry asks another. A meal made from intact foods, adequate protein, and some effortful eating often produces a different metabolic and behavioral experience than a shelf-stable snack built from refined flour, added fats, high flavor intensity, and almost no resistance. Both may contain calories. But they do not arrive with the same fullness, the same stopping power, or the same likelihood of becoming background intake.

That does not mean all refined foods have equal effects, or that every person responds identically. It means the pattern is visible enough to be explained without pretending that every calorie behaves the same once it enters a real life.

Then there is portion size.

People tend to eat more when more is put in front of them. That is not evidence of unusual weakness. It is ordinary human behavior. Larger portions shift perception. They change what feels normal, what feels satisfying, and what feels like value. When a culture steadily increases serving sizes, promotes upsizing, sells “share” packages that are routinely consumed by one person, and turns restaurant plates into oversized calorie delivery systems, intake predictably rises.

Portion creep is one of the quietest features of the modern food environment, which is one reason it is so powerful. It does not shout. It recalibrates. The wrapper grows. The cup gets taller. The default side gets larger. The bakery item becomes more like a meal. The snack becomes more like dessert. The dessert becomes large enough to be a group event and yet still lands in ordinary individual use. After enough repetition, a genuinely modest portion starts to look disappointing rather than normal.

This matters clinically because the eye learns from repetition. Appetite does too.

If a child grows up seeing oversized cups, giant muffins, restaurant plates that could feed more than one person, and a constant stream of treats framed as small indulgences, that child's sense of ordinary is being shaped before any formal nutrition lesson begins. The same is true for adults. We do not judge volume in a vacuum. We judge it against what we keep seeing.

And what we keep seeing has changed.

So has the rhythm of eating.

For much of human history, and even for much of recent history, eating was more clearly organized around meals. Not perfectly. Not universally. But more often than now, there were natural stopping points. The meal was prepared, served, eaten, and ended. The food was not always with you. It was not in every hallway, every checkout lane, every meeting room, every cupholder, every sports tournament, every waiting area, every late-night app, every drive-through lane, and every desk drawer.

That is no longer true.

Modern culture has not merely increased what people eat. It has increased how often the opportunity to eat appears. Food has become ambient. It is everywhere, and it is increasingly designed to be consumed anywhere. In line, in traffic, during email, between patients, after practice, at the movies, at the airport gate, during a conference, at the gas station, in bed, while scrolling, while driving, while barely paying attention.

Snacking is no longer just a small bridge between meals. In much of the modern food economy, it is a business model.

Natural stopping points have been designed out of the day.

A meal used to end because it ended. A pan had to be put away. A dish had to be cleared. A kitchen had to be reopened for the next episode of food. Those are forms of friction. Modern food culture often removes them. Resealable packages, individually wrapped products, shelf-stable snacks, large beverage containers, delivery apps, and foods designed for one-handed eating all make continuation easier. They reduce the pauses in which the body might have asked, with some authority, whether more was really needed.

Friction is an underrated metabolic ally.

Not because life should be made harder for people, but because some kinds of friction protect against mindless excess. Washing produce is friction. Cooking protein is friction. Sitting down for a meal is friction. Plating food is friction. Even the perishability of whole foods can be protective, because it limits how long and how casually they can remain in the environment. When friction disappears entirely, the body is often left trying to regulate intake in a setting that has been meticulously organized against pause.

Not all friction is good. The book's larger argument is that we should reduce the friction that makes healthier eating hard. But we should be honest that eliminating all friction from eating does not produce wisdom. It often produces more consumption.

That is one reason convenience must be discussed carefully. Convenience itself is not the villain. For working families, caregivers, shift workers, parents with long commutes, students, and people living with financial stress, convenience can be the difference between eating and not eating. It can make survival possible. Criticizing convenience from a distance is one of the easiest mistakes a comfortable observer can make.

The deeper problem is that the most convenient options in the current system are too often the ones that are easiest to overconsume.

We built convenience in a way that often travels with low satiety, high reward, fast intake, large portions, and weak stopping points. That is the issue. Not that human beings are busy. Not that a mother buys frozen foods after a long day. Not that a worker grabs something packaged between obligations. The issue is that a great deal of what the system offers those people has been engineered to solve time and shelf-life problems while quietly worsening metabolic ones.

Put more bluntly: we did not just make food faster. We often made it easier to overeat.

That helps explain why education alone loses so often against exposure.

If information alone were enough, the most informed society in history would not be struggling this badly. Public health messaging has sometimes behaved as though information were the decisive variable. Teach people the basics. Show them the label. Explain calories. Explain sugar. Explain portion size. Some of that matters. People deserve clear information. But information is a weak force when it must fight an environment that is constant, sensory, cheap, visible, and embedded in routine.

Education is a voice.

Exposure is a chorus.

A person may know perfectly well what a healthier choice would be and still arrive at 8:30 p.m. under-slept, behind schedule, low on patience, with children still to feed and a refrigerator that does not yet resemble a fresh-food fantasy. In that moment, knowledge is still present. It is simply outnumbered. Exposure has the sensory appeal. Exposure has the convenience. Exposure has the speed. Exposure often has the lower immediate cost, the longer shelf life, and the easier cleanup. Exposure has been rehearsing its argument since the commute home.

Even clinicians are not exempt from that reality. A physician can understand metabolic disease professionally and still feel the pull of the vending machine on a long shift. A dietitian can know precisely how satiety works and still find late-night ultra-processed snacks strangely persuasive under fatigue. Knowledge does not remove physiology. It does not erase stress. It does not make a highly engineered food environment stop behaving like one.

This is why shame is such a poor teacher in obesity care.

Shame assumes the person simply did not know enough or did not care enough. But many people struggling with weight know more than the culture gives them credit for. They may know a great deal and still be losing, day after day, to exposure that is more persistent than their ability to resist it indefinitely. The right response to that is not contempt. It is a better map.

A better map recognizes that the question cannot be only, "What did you choose?"

The better question is also, "What kept being put in front of you?"

In what package. In what portion. At what hour. After what kind of day. At what price. In what state of fatigue. With what alternatives actually available.

Once the question changes, the field of responsibility widens.

If a large fraction of the food supply is engineered around convenience, repeated appeal, fast intake, and long shelf life, then obesity becomes understandable not only as a matter of personal behavior, but as a predictable downstream effect of food design. Much of the epidemic can be understood through food engineering, not just food ignorance. That does not mean every company intended to create disease. It means the system has rewarded products whose advantages in storage, transport, cost, and consumer appeal also happen to align dangerously well with overconsumption.

That is a harder truth than "people should know better."

It is also a more useful one.

Because once we understand the problem as design, new questions become possible. Why are highly processed products so dominant in some settings? Why are they often the most durable, visible, and aggressively marketed? Why do convenience, affordability, and metabolic quality so often pull in opposite directions? Why are healthier defaults so often harder to find in the moments when people are most depleted? Why does medicine spend so much time documenting the downstream complications of a food environment it still rarely has the power to meaningfully interrupt?

Those questions belong to the chapters ahead. But the processed-food argument has to land first, because without it the whole discussion stays too abstract. Obesity is not only about weak choices confronting good information. It is also about a food system that has become very good at making calorie delivery easy, rewarding, portable, and nearly continuous.

And if that sounds too strong, consider how ordinary the evidence has become. Walk the average airport. Walk the average convenience store. Walk the center aisles of the average supermarket. Open the average office snack drawer. Watch what is marketed at children. Watch what appears at eye level near the register. Notice what can sit for months, what can be opened with one hand, what can be eaten in a car, what can be sold cheaply in large quantities, and what is framed not as a special occasion but as daily life.

The food supply does not merely sit there waiting for wise consumers to navigate it. It presents, cues, nudges, reminds, stimulates, and normalizes. It teaches appetite what to expect. It teaches the eye what looks ordinary. It teaches the day to contain more eating moments than the body was ever asked to manage in calmer conditions.

In that sense, the modern food supply does more than feed people.

It trains patterns that make excess intake easier to repeat.

That sentence needs one final layer of care, because the book's argument is not that every person eating ultra-processed food is doing something reckless, or that every household can simply opt out tomorrow. Many families are operating inside tight budgets, tight schedules, neighborhoods with limited healthier-food access, transportation constraints, caregiving burdens, and energy limits that make the current marketplace feel less like a menu and more like a trap. The critique here is not directed at people using the system. It is directed at the system that keeps offering them the same metabolically difficult bargain.

Cheap, easy, engineered calories now do too much of the heavy lifting in daily American eating. They arrive with less preparation, less spoilage, less waiting, and often less immediate cost than the foods most likely to support satiety, body composition, and long-term health. That arrangement did not appear by accident. It was built.

And what is built can be rebuilt.

That does not require fantasy. It does not require abolishing pleasure, packaged food, industry, or convenience. It requires a more serious target. It requires asking whether convenience can be paired with nourishment instead of routinely paired with passive overconsumption. It requires asking whether portion norms, product formulation, placement, school food, workplace food, retail design, and benefit design can do more to support a metabolically healthier default. It requires asking whether physicians, public health leaders, insurers, educators, and business leaders are willing to confront not only what people eat, but what the system keeps making easiest to eat.

Those are upstream questions.

They matter because downstream treatment, however important, will always be forced to work harder if the intake side of the equation is being trained in the wrong direction from morning until night. Medication can help. Surgery can help. Counseling can help. They all matter. But if food engineering keeps lowering the friction of overconsumption while daily life keeps thinning the time and energy available for self-regulation, the rescue system will always be chasing a moving target.

The modern food environment did not merely make calories available.

It made them easy to continue.

This chapter has focused on design: the taste, form, texture, speed, size, and ubiquity of the foods now surrounding people. But design is only part of the story. These products did not become dominant only because they are rewarding. They became dominant because they also fit the economics of modern life. They store well. They travel well. They scale well. They often cost less per calorie. They are easy for business models to distribute and for strapped households to rely on.

To understand why the foods most engineered for overconsumption are so often the foods most practical to buy, we have to follow the incentives from the package to the pocketbook.

That is where we turn next.

Chapter Four: The Cheap-Calorie Economy

The package and the pocketbook are closer than they look.

It is late in the week, and the grocery cart is being pushed by arithmetic.

A parent moves through the store with a rough budget in mind, a tired body, and the clear knowledge that dinner still has to happen tonight. Chicken would be useful. Berries look good. Salad would feel like the kind of choice a doctor would approve of. But some of it is expensive for what it provides, some of it may spoil, and all of it asks for time that may or may not still exist by the time the family gets home. A few aisles over are foods that cost less up front, last longer, survive rough handling, and can feed hungry people fast.

In that moment, the contest is not between virtue and vice.

It is between what is biologically wiser and what the week makes doable.

This is one of the least understood forces in the obesity story. We often talk as if the main struggle were between knowledge and temptation, or between discipline and indulgence. But for millions of people, a large part of the struggle is economic. Cheap, convenient calories are often easier to buy, easier to store, easier to transport, easier to serve, and easier to live on than the foods most likely to support satiety, body composition, and long-term metabolic health.

That does not mean families are foolish. It means they are adapting to the terms in front of them.

When money is tight, time is thin, and the household still has to be fed, one brutal measure starts to matter more than people like to admit: how much usable energy can be purchased for the money available. In that contest, refined starches, added sugars, inexpensive oils, and heavily processed foods can be fierce competitors. They can deliver a lot of calories at low cost. They can quiet hunger quickly. They can stretch a budget in the short term.

That is not the only way food should be judged. It may not even be the best way. But scarcity changes the scoreboard.

Food debates become confused because different people are playing by different rules. A physician may be thinking about protein, blood sugar, fiber, nutrient density, and long-term disease risk. A parent in a grocery aisle may be thinking about dollars left until payday, whether the food will survive the week, whether the children will actually eat it, and whether there will be enough time and energy to prepare it after work tomorrow. Both are thinking about reality. But the realities are not the same.

The modern food economy has become extraordinarily efficient at manufacturing calories. It has been less consistent at delivering satiety, protein adequacy, nutrient density, and freshness with the same ease and price. That matters because bodies do not merely need energy. They need food that helps regulate appetite, preserve muscle, support health, and remain livable in ordinary life.

An honest argument has to pause here.

Not every healthier food is expensive. Beans, lentils, oats, potatoes, eggs, plain yogurt, canned fish, frozen vegetables, peanut butter, and other practical staples can be cost-conscious, useful foods. Many families build strong meals around them every day. It would be lazy, and untrue, to pretend that the only alternative to ultra-processed eating is expensive produce, boutique groceries, or restaurant-level spending.

But that truth, important as it is, does not erase the larger problem.

People do not eat one heroic ingredient at a time. They live whole weeks.

A bag of dry beans may be affordable. So may oats. So may eggs. But a real life still has to absorb the shopping, the storage, the cooking, the cleanup, the repetition, and the uncertainty. A household does not need one photographable healthy meal. It needs an eating pattern that can survive Monday, Tuesday, Thursday night traffic, a sick child, an unexpectedly late shift, a low-fridge evening, and the ordinary fatigue that makes one more task feel larger than it looks on paper.

That is why the price of food is not only the number on the label.

Price is also what the food asks of your life.

Does it ask for chopping, cooking, and cleanup? Does it ask for a working kitchen, a freezer with room, or another trip to the store in three days? Does it ask for planning that begins the night before? Does it ask the shopper to gamble against spoilage? Does it ask for a calm evening that may never arrive? The register records the dollars. It does not record the time, the transport, the refrigeration, the kitchen equipment, the attention, or the emotional bandwidth.

Two foods can look similar in price and feel very different in cost.

A package that can sit in a pantry for weeks carries one kind of cost. A fresh food that asks to be used soon carries another. A drive-through meal is not only selling calories. It is selling relief. A boxed snack is not only selling taste. It is selling predictability. In a crowded life, that matters.

Sometimes what people are buying is not merely food.

They are buying escape from one more task.

This is one reason cheap calories keep winning. Cheap calories are not only cheap. They are forgiving.

A bag of chips does not wilt. A box of crackers does not turn brown. A package of snack cakes does not punish the household because soccer ran late on Tuesday and work ran late on Wednesday. A sweetened beverage can wait in the refrigerator. A frozen pizza can sit for weeks as insurance against a day that falls apart. Fresh berries can mold. Greens can collapse in the crisper drawer. Fish asks for a plan. Chicken asks for one too. Cut produce asks to be used soon. For a household with little room for waste, long shelf life is not a small advantage. It is a form of security.

Waste is expensive.

That is easy to forget from the outside. But when money is tight, throwing out spoiled produce or unused fresh food does not feel like a minor disappointment. It feels like money lost to a system that already asks too much. Under those conditions, shelf-stable foods start to look responsible, not reckless. Families are not necessarily optimizing for perfect metabolic health in those moments. More often, they are optimizing against waste, against uncertainty, and against the chaos of a week that may not cooperate.

Transport and storage matter too.

If the nearest full grocery store is not close, if the trip happens by bus, if the car is unreliable, if the refrigerator is small, if the freezer is crowded, or if the household cannot easily shop twice a week, then foods that travel well and survive the week start looking not just convenient but rational. Families do not choose inside an ideal marketplace. They choose inside transportation limits, storage limits, time limits, and cash-flow limits.

That burden does not fall evenly.

The more constrained a household is by money, schedule volatility, transport, neighborhood food access, and kitchen stability, the more power the cheap-calorie economy tends to have. This is not because some families care less about health. It is because healthier eating often requires buffer, and scarcity strips away buffer first.

Buffer money to shop before the pantry is nearly empty. Buffer time to cook. Buffer refrigeration space. Buffer energy to wash, chop, and try again tomorrow. Buffer attention to plan ahead. Buffer flexibility to recover from a spoiled carton of berries or a meal nobody would eat. Healthy eating often asks for more buffer than the culture admits. Many people are living with very little of it.

Businesses notice the same realities.

Products that travel well, resist spoilage, stack neatly, sit on shelves, and still look sellable days or weeks later are easier to scale than foods that bruise, rot, leak, demand refrigeration, or expire quickly. Fresh strawberries and leafy greens are living biological goods. Chips, cookies, sweetened cereals, packaged desserts, and many snack foods are logistical goods. One category asks the retailer to manage waste carefully. The other is built for warehousing, display, and repeat sale.

This is not an anti-grocer argument.

Retailers live inside math. A product that survives shipping, fills an endcap, tolerates delayed purchase, and looks identical from one week to the next carries commercial advantages that a peach does not. A case of soda can be stacked, promoted, and discounted in a way that fresh spinach cannot. Shelf-stable products usually tolerate the business system more easily than fragile foods do. The problem is not that merchants understand margin. The problem is that the larger market often rewards durability, convenience, and repeat purchase more reliably than it rewards nutrient quality.

The food economy is not morally confused because it is an economy. It is doing what incentive systems do. It is moving toward what stores well, sells reliably, creates value perception, and can be distributed at scale.

That is why cheap calories win so often. They solve several problems at once.

They solve the money problem by delivering a lot of energy for relatively little cash. They solve the storage problem by lasting. They solve the time problem by asking for little preparation. They solve the uncertainty problem by being familiar and reliable. They often solve the child-acceptance problem better than more labor-intensive meals do. And because they are so available, they solve the immediate hunger problem fast.

The problem is not that any one of those features is evil. The problem is that together they create a market advantage for foods that often work against metabolic health.

A great deal of public advice collapses under this reality.

"Just buy healthier food" sounds reasonable only if one imagines an ideal shopper with stable income, reliable transport, a functioning kitchen, room in the refrigerator, time to cook, confidence that the food will not be wasted, and enough household calm to carry a plan through the week. Many people are not shopping under those conditions.

Just buy healthier food with what cash flow?

With what extra store trip?

With what confidence that the produce will still be good on Friday?

With what kitchen time after the commute, the homework, the laundry, the email, the dishes, and the hour of evening already spoken for?

With what backup plan if work runs late again tomorrow?

A person standing in that reality is not choosing between perfect health and negligence. More often, that person is choosing between what is ideal and what is executable.

That distinction matters morally as much as it matters medically.

If you have ever stood in a grocery aisle or a checkout line with too little time, a tight budget, and a family still to feed, then you know how quickly food advice can begin to sound like judgment when it ignores the life in which it must be followed. The phrase "just eat better" lands very differently when the week is already operating at its edge.

This is where medicine has often underpriced effort.

Clinicians mean well when they encourage more home cooking, more fresh food, more meal planning, more protein, more produce, fewer packaged snacks, fewer sugary drinks. Much of that advice is biologically sound. But advice becomes thin when it underestimates the commercial and practical environment patients are being asked to overcome. We can accidentally speak as though better eating were merely a matter of wanting it badly enough, when in reality it may require more time, more money, more predictability, and more daily labor than the household currently has.

Good advice can still fail if execution costs too much.

That is one of the crueler aspects of the modern obesity story. We often ask the people under the most financial and time pressure to perform the most expensive version of adherence. We ask them to buy foods that may be pricier in useful forms, require more preparation, spoil more easily, and compete poorly against cheaper, faster, highly visible alternatives. Then we are tempted to interpret the struggle as insufficient motivation.

But adherence does not happen in the abstract.

It happens in kitchens, stores, cars, break rooms, corner shops, drive-through lanes, vending areas, and late evenings.

The grocery store is one of the clearest places to see the mismatch between clinic logic and market logic.

In the exam room, the message is often straightforward: favor protein, vegetables, fruit, higher-fiber foods, and less processed eating. Reduce sugary drinks. Eat with more structure. Try not to let every snack become a meal and every meal become a delivery system for cheap excess calories.

Then the patient leaves.

The marketplace speaks in a different voice. Value-size packages promise more for less. Promotional displays offer large amounts of processed food at eye level. Sweetened beverages are sold cold, cheap, and ready. Packaged snack foods can be bought in bulk and stored as backup. Checkout lanes rehearse impulse. Foods that require almost no preparation gather around the tired hour of the day like a practical solution, because in many ways they are one.

The exam room gives advice for minutes.

The marketplace gives counter-advice all week.

This does not make the grocery store evil. It makes it revealing. The store is a map of incentives. It places before people what sells, what stores, what moves with margin, what suppliers support, what shoppers under pressure reliably choose, and what can survive the long logistics of modern retail. Health may be one value in that system. It is not usually the only one, and often not the strongest one.

The same pattern extends well beyond the supermarket.

It appears in gas stations, vending machines, airport kiosks, office snack tables, school concessions, pharmacies, dollar menus, and convenience stores. The common feature is not one company or one aisle. The common feature is the repeated pairing of ease, durability, and fast energy. The foods most available in the moments when people are busiest, most depleted, or farthest from a kitchen are often the foods least likely to support good metabolic health over time.

That repeated pairing leaves a mark.

When people live for years inside an environment where cheap, durable, ready-to-eat calories are the most reliable answer to the most exhausted moments of the day, the body begins receiving the same message over and over. Not only that food is available, but that the easiest food will usually be the most processed, the most portable, and the least demanding of time. A culture can get very good at feeding people quickly while quietly becoming poor at feeding them well.

Convenience deserves more respect in this conversation than it usually gets.

Too often convenience is treated as a polite word for laziness. It is not. Convenience is one of the hidden forces shaping metabolic health. A meal that can be heated in minutes, eaten by tired children without an argument, and cleaned up quickly has genuine value in a strained household. A food that can wait in the pantry until the schedule collapses has strategic value. A drive-through window can feel like rescue at 8:00 p.m., not indulgence. All of that is real.

The problem is not that people need convenience.

The problem is that the convenience tier of the modern food system is too often built from cheap, highly processed calories that are easy to overconsume and hard to build long-term health around.

Healthy convenience does exist. Greek yogurt. Hard-boiled eggs. Rotisserie chicken. Frozen vegetables. Pre-washed greens. Ready beans. Canned fish. Higher-protein meals. Fruit that travels well. Better freezer options. These can help. They matter. But the healthier convenience layer is often thinner, less visible, less aggressively promoted, or more expensive than the calorie-dense alternatives surrounding it. The competition is not always fair.

If two foods were equally available, equally affordable, equally ready, equally accepted by the household, and equally easy to repeat, the healthier one would often have a much better chance.

But they are not offered on equal terms.

That is the hidden force.

By the time many people are making food decisions, they are not spending only money. They are spending judgment. A food that asks one minute and almost no thought is competing against a food that asks ten or twenty minutes, several decisions, some kitchen work, and cleanup. The difference is not merely culinary. It is cognitive. Decision fatigue changes what feels possible, and the market is full of foods designed to appear as low-friction answers to high-friction days.

The language of value makes this harder.

The marketplace has taught people, understandably, to associate value with more ounces, bigger portions, larger cups, extra servings, family-size packages, combo deals, and bulk purchase. In tight financial conditions, that can sound like responsibility. Sometimes it is responsibility, in the narrow sense of buying enough food to get through the week. But the body's definition of value is not identical to the market's. The body values protein, fiber, slower intake, better satiety, preserved muscle, and useful nourishment. The market often highlights quantity first.

So a family can be nudged toward more calories in the name of thrift.

That is not because the family is irrational. It is because the bargain is framed around immediate volume, not long-term metabolic outcomes. A larger sugary drink, a bigger bag, a two-for-one dessert, a family-size snack box, a larger side for little extra money. The economy is teaching a lesson, and the lesson is usually about abundance per dollar.

The receipt, of course, is not the whole bill.

The same food that is cheap in the aisle can be expensive in the body if it repeatedly drives excess intake, weakens nutrient density, worsens blood sugar, displaces protein, disrupts satiety, and contributes over time to the long list of downstream complications medicine then has to treat. The tragedy is that the bills are paid in different places. One is paid today at the register. The other is paid later in the clinic, the pharmacy, the sleep lab, the imaging center, and the ordinary fatigue of daily life.

A system can therefore look cheap while being expensive.

That is part of what makes this chapter so important. The modern diet is not merely a story about preference. It is a story about pricing, perishability, packaging, logistics, retail design, and the daily economics of fatigue. People are not only eating what tastes good. They are eating what fits the timetable, the household budget, the pantry, the commute, and the amount of life left in them by the time food has to be chosen.

Once that becomes visible, the obesity conversation changes.

It becomes harder to say that people simply need more information. It becomes harder to say that better individual choice, by itself, is a complete answer. It becomes harder to ignore the commercial structure that keeps making cheap, durable calories easier to live on than the foods most likely to support health.

And it becomes harder to dismiss healthy-food access as some optional lifestyle concern floating outside real medicine.

When the friction of eating well is built into price, transport, storage, time, and convenience, access is no longer a side issue. It becomes part of the clinical picture. A patient can understand every word of good nutrition advice and still find that the environment keeps charging extra for living by it. That extra charge may come in dollars, or it may come in time, planning, spoilage risk, and decision fatigue. Either way, the cost is real.

This is not a call to romanticize the past, shame working families, or pretend that every packaged food is the enemy. It is a call to tell the truth about the present.

The truth is that modern households often do not buy food inside an ideal marketplace.

They buy food inside time pressure.

Inside uncertainty.

Inside fatigue.

Inside a commercial system that has become exceptionally skilled at making cheap, durable calories easy to obtain.

That truth should change the posture of obesity medicine. It should make us slower to judge and quicker to understand execution barriers. It should make us more serious about the economics of food access. It should make us less impressed with advice that sounds correct in theory but ignores the daily math of the people expected to follow it. And it should make us willing to say that the modern diet is not just a nutritional problem.

It is an economic design problem.

A cheap-calorie economy strains all four lines of the model at once. It makes calorie excess easier. It often makes protein adequacy harder to protect. It weakens nutrient density. And because the environment keeps steering the day toward what is cheap, durable, and fast, it makes adherence harder to sustain.

That is what the marketplace is doing before the clinic ever sees the lab results.

Healthcare will continue to spend enormous effort on what this economy helps create. Some of that work is noble and necessary. But if obesity medicine wants to think clearly, it has to see the supermarket, the pantry, the vending machine, the gas station, and the drive-through as part of the clinical story. Not because medicine should control dinner. Because dinner has already been influencing the clinic for years.

Even so, weight alone is still too crude a way to understand what the body is carrying.

The cheap-calorie economy helps explain why body weight rises so easily in modern life. But the number on the scale does not tell us the whole story. It does not tell us how much of that weight is fat, how much is muscle, how much function has been lost, or how well the body is actually being supported.

To care well for obesity, we have to move beyond pounds alone.

We have to ask a more precise question: what is the body made of, and what does that mean for health?

Chapter Five: Weight Is Not the Same as Health

For many people, the scale has become a kind of courtroom.

A person steps onto it in a clinic, at a pharmacy, in a gym corner, or at home before getting dressed, and waits for a number that seems to say much more than gravity. Sometimes that number can shape the mood of a whole day. It can feel like news, judgment, confession, or failure before any better question has even been asked.

That feeling did not come from nowhere. The culture has spent decades teaching people to treat pounds as if they were the cleanest summary of health. Smaller is assumed to mean better. Larger is assumed to mean worse. The body is reduced to one figure, and that figure is asked to carry far more meaning than it can honestly hold.

But if the scale is going to carry that much authority, it should at least be precise enough for the job.

It is not.

The last chapters helped explain why body weight can rise so easily in modern life. Cheap, engineered, convenient calories can push intake upward while making regulation harder. That part matters. But once weight has gone up, the next question is not merely how high the number is. The next question is what that number represents.

The scale measures total load.

It does not sort the cargo.

It cannot tell how much of a person's weight is body fat, how much is muscle, how much is water, and how much is simple short-term fluctuation. It cannot tell whether a salty meal, a long trip, a hard workout, poor sleep, hormonal shifts, or the timing of yesterday's meals changed the number. It cannot tell whether the body is becoming more capable or less capable. It can record motion. It cannot explain meaning.

That matters because two people can weigh the same and have very different bodies. They can carry different amounts of body fat, different amounts of muscle, different levels of physical function, and different levels of metabolic risk. They can live in very different physiology while sharing a number.

Two people can also lose the same amount of weight and not arrive at the same outcome at all. One may reduce excess body fat while preserving strength, mobility, and health. Another may lose a good deal of useful lean tissue, feel weaker, and become less resilient in the process. The scale gives both stories the same headline.

The body bears the difference.

This is where obesity medicine has to become more serious than the culture. The public conversation often treats body size as if it were the whole story. Better medicine cannot afford that shortcut.

Weight matters. It is not meaningless. Large changes in body weight can reflect very real biological change, and excess body weight can matter both mechanically and metabolically. But weight alone is still too blunt an instrument to define health, guide treatment, or tell a person what kind of progress is actually taking place.

The more precise medical question is not simply, How much does the body weigh?

It is, How much excess body fat is present, where is it stored, what is it doing to the body, and how well is the body still functioning?

That is a very different question.

Doctors use the word adiposity to mean body fat. In careful obesity medicine, obesity is not best understood as vaguely “weighing too much.” It is better understood as excess adiposity in an amount or pattern that is burdening health, impairing function, or increasing risk in a meaningful way.

That language is more accurate. It is also more humane.

It moves the conversation away from appearance and toward biology. It shifts the focus from how a person looks to what the tissue is doing, where it is being carried, what complications may be emerging, and what burden it is placing on daily life. That is a better frame for science, and it is a better frame for dignity.

Body fat is not just passive padding. It is living tissue. In the wrong amount and the wrong places, it can push blood sugar, blood pressure, liver health, sleep quality, inflammation, and the body's handling of hunger in the wrong direction. It can also burden the body mechanically. Joints may hurt. Breathing during sleep may worsen. Reflux may worsen. Stamina may fall. The work of carrying the body through ordinary life can become harder.

None of that is a character flaw.

It is physiology.

It is also why obesity should never be treated as a purely cosmetic concern. The issue is not that bodies must conform to some visual ideal. The issue is that excess adiposity can alter health from the inside and strain function from the outside. A person may experience that through rising blood sugar, fatty liver, worsening sleep apnea, high blood pressure, worsening mobility, increasing pain, or a long list of other complications that have nothing to do with aesthetics.

Function deserves much more respect in this conversation than it usually gets. Can the body rise from a chair easily? Climb stairs without marked breathlessness? Walk through an airport, carry groceries, sleep well, recover from illness, and move through the day with some reserve instead of constant strain? These are not cosmetic questions. They are health questions.

Performance, in this sense, does not mean athletic excellence. It means everyday human capability.

It means being able to live in the body with more freedom and less burden.

That is one reason weight alone can be so misleading. A person can weigh less and function worse. A person can lose weight and unintentionally lose too much of the tissue that was helping them remain strong, independent, and metabolically protected. Another person may lose less weight than expected while making real gains in blood sugar, sleep, mobility, waist size, stamina, and quality of life.

The culture notices pounds first.

The body notices everything.

This is the point at which body composition becomes essential.

Body composition means what the body is made of. In plain language, how much of the body is body fat and how much is lean tissue, including muscle and other non-fat tissue. That distinction matters because health is influenced not only by how heavy the body is, but by what kind of tissue the body is carrying.

Lean tissue matters. Muscle matters. It matters for movement, balance, strength, recovery, glucose handling, and long-term independence. It matters when someone gets up from the floor, climbs stairs, lifts a child, carries bags from the car, or tries to recover from surgery, illness, or just an exhausting week. A body with less excess fat and preserved muscle is not the same as a body that became smaller by sacrificing too much strength along the way.

Yet the public conversation often treats all weight loss as if it were automatically the same kind of victory.

It is not.

A person can become lighter because of careful treatment, improved food structure, preserved protein intake, and improving health. A person can also become lighter because of under-eating, illness, grief, medication side effects, dehydration, or loss of useful lean tissue. The scale does not know the difference unless medicine asks it.

That is why “goal weight” is an incomplete concept when used by itself. It may still have some use. But if the goal is defined only as a smaller number, people can be congratulated for changes that leave them weaker, more fatigued, or less well nourished than before. The culture often praises weight loss before asking what was lost.

That is not careful enough.

This is also where one of the most familiar tools in medicine needs more humility.

BMI, or body mass index, is a ratio based on weight and height. It is quick. It is cheap. It is easy to calculate, which is one reason healthcare systems and public health discussions use it so often. Across large populations, it can be useful as a rough screening tool. It can help raise a flag that more evaluation may be needed.

But BMI is not a body-composition scan.

It cannot tell whether the weight comes mostly from body fat, mostly from muscle, or from some mix of body fat, muscle, bone, and fluid. It does not tell where fat is stored. It does not tell whether a person is strong or frail. It does not tell whether blood sugar is already rising, whether the liver is filling with fat, whether sleep apnea is present, or whether the knees and back are increasingly carrying more burden than they can comfortably tolerate.

BMI can open the chart.

It cannot close the case.

A muscular person can fall into a BMI category that sounds alarming without carrying the same degree of metabolic risk as someone whose extra weight is made up of far more body fat. An older adult can have a BMI that appears unremarkable while carrying too little muscle, too much abdominal fat, and far more metabolic vulnerability than the number suggests. A person can be in a weight range often viewed as socially acceptable and still have increased liver fat, insulin resistance, low fitness, and worsening sleep. Another can live at a higher weight and have a different pattern of complications, function, and risk than the stereotype would predict.

None of that means BMI is useless.

It means BMI is incomplete.

A rough population tool becomes dangerous when it is mistaken for a complete individual diagnosis.

That distinction is important in both directions. It protects people at higher weights from lazy judgments that pretend a number tells the whole story. And it protects people at lower weights from false reassurance that says everything must be fine because the number does not look alarming.

Precision protects both directions.

Part of what makes this chapter necessary is that the body does not store fat identically in every person. Location matters.

Some body fat sits mostly under the skin. Some is stored deeper in the abdomen, around the organs. That deeper abdominal fat is often called visceral fat. Readers do not need to memorize the term to understand the problem. Fat stored deep around the organs tends to behave differently than fat stored more superficially. It is more closely linked to insulin resistance, fatty liver, abnormal blood fats, and the cluster of metabolic problems that so often travel together.

This is one reason a tape measure can sometimes tell a truth the scale misses.

Waist size is not the whole story either. But it can reveal central fat accumulation that body weight by itself does not describe well. A person can weigh less than expected and still carry too much risk in the abdomen and liver. Another can weigh more than expected and carry a different balance of risk than the culture assumes at first glance.

Again, nuance does not mean denial.

It does not mean excess body fat suddenly stops mattering.

It means where fat is carried, what kind of tissue is being protected, and what complications are present all matter too.

A body can also be metabolically struggling before the mirror gives anyone permission to worry. That is one reason appearance is such a poor clinical tool. It can miss deeper fat around the abdomen and organs. It can miss declining muscle. It can miss rising blood sugar, fatty liver, and sleep-disordered breathing that are already changing a person's health long before the culture decides they "look" sick enough to count.

This is why serious obesity medicine has to ask better questions than the culture usually asks. Not only, What is the weight? But also, What is the waist? What is the blood sugar doing? What is the liver doing? What is happening to blood pressure, sleep, stamina, mobility, pain, and day-to-day capability? How much muscle is being preserved? Is the body becoming easier to live in, or harder?

Those questions produce a richer and more truthful picture than pounds alone.

They also produce a kinder one.

No clinic needs perfect technology to start thinking more clearly. A careful history helps. A waist measurement helps. Blood pressure helps. Blood work helps. Questions about sleep, movement, stamina, pain, and day-to-day function help. When body-composition tools are available, they can add detail. But precision begins with asking better questions, not with owning the fanciest machine.

Stigma thrives in crude conversations. When a culture talks as if body size were a simple moral summary of a person, people get judged before they get understood. They get reduced to appearance. They get lectured when they need evaluation. They get offered simplistic advice for a problem that is far more biologically and socially complicated than the lecture implies.

Precision interrupts that.

When medicine becomes more precise, it also becomes more humane.

A person living with obesity is no longer reduced to appearance or a number on a chart. The discussion shifts to excess adiposity, tissue quality, fat distribution, mechanical burden, metabolic burden, sleep, function, and complications. That is not colder language. It is more respectful language. It gives the person back some individuality. It lowers the chance that the whole conversation will collapse into appearance and blame.

At the same time, precision protects us from another mistake: pretending that common disease is normal health. If a person is developing fatty liver, worsening blood sugar, sleep apnea, high blood pressure, joint strain, or declining function, denial does not become compassion just because the condition is common. Bodies still pay the price. The answer is not to soften the science until no one feels uncomfortable. The answer is to tell the truth without humiliating people.

This chapter sits inside that tension on purpose.

Respect and truth have to stay together.

A better definition of obesity helps with that. It tells us that obesity is not a beauty judgment. It is not a personality type. It is not a synonym for laziness. It is a clinical condition involving excess adiposity and its consequences. Those consequences can vary from person to person. They can be metabolic, mechanical, functional, or several at once. But once we understand the condition that way, the conversation becomes more anchored in reality and less contaminated by stereotype.

That change matters for treatment too. If a clinician is focused only on the scale, treatment goals become narrow very quickly. The whole enterprise can collapse into pounds lost per month. But if the clinician is focused on body composition, fat distribution, function, and complications, the goals become more intelligent. We start caring not only about whether the number moved, but whether the person is preserving strength, improving blood sugar, sleeping better, reducing liver fat, moving more freely, and becoming more resilient.

Those are the kinds of outcomes people actually live inside.

They are also the outcomes that make a body healthier even before dramatic visible change occurs.

A person may not look profoundly different after several months of careful treatment. But the waist may be down. Blood sugar may be better. Sleep may be safer. Energy may be steadier. Pain may be lower. Function may be improving. The liver may be under less strain. The body may be moving in a better direction long before the culture decides to approve of what it sees.

That is one reason people deserve better than scale-centered thinking. It is too narrow for science and too harsh for human beings.

We have become a scale-literate culture, but not yet a body-composition-literate one.

We know how to react to pounds.

We are less practiced at asking what those pounds are made of, where risk is concentrated, what function is being gained or lost, and what kind of health the body is actually building.

Healthcare has contributed to that problem. A quick number fits easily into a chart, a waiting room flow, a public-health dashboard, and a wellness program. A more complete understanding asks more of the visit. It asks for clinical attention, better questions, better tools, and more humility. But serious fields do not earn the right to stay crude just because crude is faster.

Obesity medicine has to be better than that.

It has to be willing to say that weight is relevant without pretending weight is the whole truth. It has to distinguish body size from body composition, appearance from disease burden, and visible change from meaningful improvement. It has to care about adiposity, where that adiposity is carried, how the person is functioning, and what complications are already emerging.

Most of all, it has to give patients a better target.

The goal is not simply to weigh less.

The goal is to carry healthier tissue, function better, and reduce disease burden.

And once that target becomes clear, the next challenge becomes unavoidable. Once we stop calling every smaller body a better body, we have to ask a more exact question.

If treatment is not just about becoming smaller, then what exactly must be protected while excess body fat is being reduced?

The answer is not mysterious.

It is muscle.

It is strength.

It is function.

That is where we turn next.

Chapter Six: Lose Fat, Keep Muscle

There is a familiar moment in obesity care that sounds like uncomplicated good news.

The number is down.

The clothes fit differently. The chart looks better. The room relaxes. A person who has been carrying years of frustration finally feels some movement in the right direction.

And yet the most important question may still be unanswered.

What, exactly, became smaller?

That question is quieter than the scale, but medically it is often more important. Weight can go down in ways that improve health, preserve strength, and reduce disease burden. Weight can also go down in ways that leave a person weaker, less capable, and less protected than before. The scale can record both stories with equal enthusiasm.

It cannot tell us which tissue paid for the victory.

That is why the second line of this book's model matters so much in real life. Quantity in calories influences body weight. But quality of macronutrient balance, especially protein adequacy, influences body composition. In plain language, the body does not only care how much was lost. The body cares what was lost.

If the last chapter asked us to move beyond pounds alone, this chapter asks a sharper question. Once treatment begins, what must be protected while excess body fat is being reduced?

The answer is muscle.

Muscle is not a cosmetic detail. It is useful tissue.

Strictly speaking, lean mass includes more than muscle. But in everyday life, muscle is the part most people need to picture when they hear the word protection. Muscle helps you rise from a chair, climb stairs, carry bags, lift children, hold balance, recover from illness, tolerate stress, and move through the ordinary demands of life with more reserve. It also helps the body handle blood sugar. It is part of metabolic health, not separate from it.

That matters because a larger body is not automatically a stronger body.

Some people living with obesity carry more weight and still have less functional muscle than the world assumes. They are carrying more load with less useful reserve. They are overburdened and underpowered at once. The culture often misses that because it keeps equating size with strength and weight loss with improvement. Real bodies are more complicated than that.

Muscle also matters because the future keeps asking something of it.

The muscle a person protects in midlife may help determine how well that person tolerates aging, injury, surgery, illness, and the slow accumulation of ordinary wear. A body that loses excess fat while keeping strength is not just changing its appearance. It is protecting its future options. It is preserving independence. It is building a better margin of safety.

This is one reason obesity treatment should never be framed as making the body smaller alone. The true aim is not simply a smaller body.

The true aim is not simply to occupy less space.

The true aim is to carry less harmful fat while preserving as much strength, function, and useful tissue as possible.

That sounds obvious once stated plainly. In practice, it is often neglected.

Weight-loss culture has trained people to celebrate subtraction first and ask questions later. The number fell. Therefore the result must be good. But biology is not that careless. When intake falls, the body does not politely read your intentions and remove only the exact tissue you would have chosen. Unless the process is structured well, some of the loss can come from places you needed to protect.

Fat loss is the target.

Muscle should not be treated as collateral damage.

This is where protein enters the story, not as a fad, not as a tribal identity, and not as a bonus for athletes, but as one of the central tools of competent obesity treatment.

Protein matters because it helps the body maintain and repair lean tissue. It also often helps with fullness. Those two properties matter more than they may seem. During weight loss, the challenge is not only to lower excess energy intake. The challenge is to do so without becoming constantly hungry, physically depleted, and biologically underprotected. Protein can help on both sides of that equation.

A meal built around adequate protein often lands differently from a meal built mostly around refined starch, added sugar, or convenience calories that vanish quickly. The person may feel steadier. Hunger may return more slowly. The next food decision may arrive with less urgency. The day may become less vulnerable to improvisation.

That is not magic.

It is structure.

Protein is often underprotected in modern eating for the same reason so much else is underprotected: life is rushed, convenience is powerful, and many common foods are built around cheap calories rather than around satiety and muscle preservation. Breakfast becomes mostly starch or is skipped entirely. Lunch is improvised. Snacking fills the gaps. Dinner is then asked to rescue the whole day.

It often cannot.

One of the quiet mistakes in weight-loss culture is treating protein as if it were optional so long as calories are low enough. But low calories alone do not tell the body what to keep. A person can create a calorie deficit and still lose tissue they needed. A person can become lighter and less robust at the same time.

That is not the full kind of progress people were promised.

This does not mean everyone needs the same eating pattern. It does not mean every meal must be engineered with obsessive precision. It does not mean powders, rigid macro calculations, or a single approved menu. People eat within budgets, schedules, family routines, food preferences, cultural traditions, and medical realities. The exact plate can look many different ways.

But the principle is durable.

If fat loss is being pursued, protein usually needs to become more visible on purpose rather than being left to chance.

For some people that means eggs, yogurt, cottage cheese, fish, chicken, turkey, tofu, tempeh, beans, lentils, lean meats, edamame, or other familiar protein foods showing up more reliably and earlier in the day. For others it means restructuring meals so that protein is not an afterthought tucked under a pile of mostly refined calories. For still others, especially when appetite is low, it means recognizing that every bite now has to work harder.

That last point is becoming more important, not less, in modern obesity treatment.

We are living in an age in which powerful medications can reduce appetite in ways many patients have never experienced before. For some people, that relief is life-changing. It deserves respect. It should not be minimized or mocked. These medications can create breathing room after years of relentless hunger and repeated frustration.

But appetite reduction is not the same thing as muscle protection.

That distinction is easy to miss because the scale may respond quickly. A person eats less. Weight falls. Everyone feels encouraged. Yet a quieter appetite can also create a quieter, poorer day of eating if no one is paying attention. Breakfast disappears. Lunch becomes a few bites. Dinner is small. Protein falls with everything else. Strength work becomes irregular because energy is lower or because the patient assumes the medication itself is doing all the important work.

The scale applauds.

The body may be less impressed.

When appetite is reduced, food quality matters more, not less. Protein matters more, not less. Treatment structure matters more, not less. In this new era, good obesity care cannot simply celebrate that someone is eating less. It has to ask what is still showing up often enough to protect the person.

This is especially important because muscle preservation does not happen through diet alone.

The body needs a second message.

It needs a reason to keep the tissue.

That is the role of resistance training.

Resistance training is a phrase that sounds larger and more intimidating than it needs to be. It does not require a bodybuilder's identity, a commercial gym membership, or a social media transformation story. In simple terms, it means asking muscles to work against some form of load. That load might come from free weights, machines, resistance bands, body-weight movements, carrying, pushing, pulling, rising from a chair, or other forms of progressive effort.

The exact tool matters less than the signal.

And the signal is clear: this tissue is still needed. Keep it.

That is why resistance training deserves a special place in obesity treatment. Walking matters. Aerobic activity matters. Stamina matters. Cardiovascular fitness matters. None of that should be dismissed. But when the treatment question is specifically how to reduce excess body fat while preserving lean tissue, resistance work does something uniquely important. It helps tell the body that strength still has a job.

During a period of weight loss, unused muscle can become easy for the body to treat as expendable. Resistance training pushes back against that. It does not guarantee perfect preservation. Nothing does. But it gives protection a better chance.

This is not punishment for a larger body.

It is protection for a changing one.

That distinction matters emotionally as much as it matters physiologically. Many readers have been exposed to exercise messaging that feels humiliating, punitive, or built around aesthetics rather than health. That is not the posture here. The point of resistance training is not to force people into a gym culture they do not recognize themselves in. The point is to help the body remain capable while fat is being reduced.

For some people that may mean formal strength sessions a few times per week. For others it may begin with more modest movements: sit-to-stands, step-ups, band work, wall pushes, light dumbbells, supervised exercise, or adapted programs that respect pain, mobility limits, age, and deconditioning. The starting point can vary widely.

The principle does not.

A serious obesity treatment plan should ask not only, “How do we lower excess body fat?” It should also ask, “How do we help this person become lighter without becoming less strong or less capable?”

That question is still too uncommon in ordinary care.

Part of the problem is cultural. We glorify rapid visible change. We are less practiced at honoring quiet, protective work. It is easier to admire pounds lost than to notice that a person is preserving leg strength, standing more easily, carrying fewer symptoms, and keeping useful tissue while the waist is shrinking. But medicine should be better than the culture at knowing what counts.

Part of the problem is structural. It is easier to hand someone a scale target than to build a treatment plan that includes protein guidance, strength work, follow-up, and realistic support. It is easier to reward quick changes in body weight than to track whether the person is becoming more functional. But easier is not the same as better.

If an obesity program never discusses protein, never asks about strength work, and never checks whether the patient is becoming weaker, it is incomplete.

That incompleteness becomes especially dangerous when rapid weight loss is celebrated without enough curiosity.

The scale is impressed by speed.

The body is more discerning.

A fast drop in body weight can look exciting, especially early on. Some of that early change may reflect shifts in water and stored carbohydrate. Some of it may reflect real fat loss. Some of it may reflect a level of restriction that the person cannot sustain or that leaves too little nutritional support for lean tissue. The faster the scale moves, the more tempting it becomes to assume the method is excellent. But speed is not the same as quality.

Rapid loss can flatter the scale while cheating the body.

It can teach the wrong lesson. It can make people believe that whatever makes the number fall fastest must be the most serious or committed approach. In reality, aggressive restriction can leave a person weak, hungry, sedentary, preoccupied with food, undernourished, and more likely to rebound later. It can produce a result that looks successful from the outside but functions poorly in daily life.

This is another reason weight loss should never be treated as a contest of sheer subtraction.

A body with less excess fat and preserved strength is a better medical outcome than a body that became dramatically lighter while also becoming less capable. A slower, steadier process that protects muscle may be medically wiser than a faster process that strips away useful tissue. The public conversation rarely says this clearly enough because the public conversation is still too attached to spectacle.

Medicine should not applaud a result the body cannot afford.

That sentence matters even more in a country growing older.

As people age, muscle becomes harder to take for granted. It is one thing to lose useful tissue in youth and assume it can be rebuilt easily. It is another to move through middle age or later life with less reserve, less stability, less strength, and less protection against injury or illness. The muscle a person loses during poorly structured weight loss is not always trivial, and it is not always easily recovered.

The body keeps the books even when the culture does not.

This is why body-composition thinking is not niche thinking. It is not a side interest for fitness enthusiasts. It is one of the clearest ways obesity medicine can distinguish itself from ordinary weight-loss culture. Better treatment does not ask only whether the body is getting smaller. It asks whether the body is being built for long-term health while excess fat is being reduced.

That means the scoreboard has to improve.

Scale weight can stay on the board. It is not useless. But it cannot be the whole board.

If body-composition tools are available, they can add helpful detail. But even without sophisticated scans, better care can ask better questions. Is the waist decreasing? Is strength holding steady or improving? Is the person rising from a chair more easily, climbing stairs with less strain, carrying the body with more freedom, improving blood sugar, sleeping better, moving more comfortably, and preserving a reasonable eating pattern? Is the pace of weight loss so aggressive that the person appears increasingly depleted? Is protein showing up with enough consistency to support the process? Is the treatment making the body more functional, not just more photogenic?

Those questions are not extras.

They are part of the real job.

This matters for patients, but it also matters for the field. Obesity medicine is entering an era of greater therapeutic power. That is good news. Patients deserve effective tools. But power can tempt a field into cruder success metrics if it is not careful. When a treatment is capable of producing substantial weight loss, the risk is that everyone begins staring even harder at the number and even less at the quality of what is changing.

That would be a mistake.

The stronger our tools become, the more disciplined our definition of success must become.

In the age of obesity medications, the second line of the model becomes more important, not less. Macronutrient balance influences body composition. That truth matters more when total intake is lower. A potent appetite-lowering medication can create the opportunity for meaningful improvement. It can also expose careless treatment structure more quickly. If the program is scale-centered, the patient may lose weight while muscle quietly slips away. If the program is body-composition-centered, the patient has a better chance of losing harmful fat while remaining strong enough to enjoy the benefit.

A quiet appetite is not a complete treatment plan.

Nor is a prescription, by itself, an obesity program.

Good prescribing in this era requires an older kind of seriousness. It requires asking what the person is actually eating, whether protein has become intentional, whether the body is being asked to do enough resistance work to justify preservation, whether the rate of change is leaving the person depleted, and whether function is improving along with the number.

If those questions are absent, then modern treatment may become more powerful without becoming more precise.

That would leave patients smaller, perhaps, but not necessarily better served.

The broader public also needs a reset here. Many people still hear the phrase weight loss and picture one thing: less body. Better obesity medicine means teaching a more exact vision. The goal is not simply less body. The goal is less harmful fat, preserved muscle, better function, better metabolic health, and a body that is easier to live in.

That is a different ambition.

It is medically better.

It is morally better too.

Because when the target becomes healthier tissue instead of smaller appearance alone, the posture of treatment changes. The conversation becomes less cosmetic and more humane. The person is no longer chasing a number just to satisfy the gaze of the culture. The person is protecting capability, reserve, and long-term health. That is a more dignified project.

So when patients ask what successful obesity treatment should really look like, the answer needs to be fuller than “the scale went down.”

A better answer sounds something like this:

Excess body fat is being reduced.

Strength is being protected.

Function is improving.

Food quality is not collapsing.

The person is becoming more capable, not merely lighter.

That is what serious treatment should aim for.

Better obesity treatment is not about becoming smaller at any cost. It is about becoming healthier, stronger, and more functional.

And yet even this more precise vision still runs into a larger problem. Knowing that muscle matters does not automatically make muscle easy to protect. Protein requires structure. Resistance training requires energy and some planning. Good treatment requires follow-through. All of that has to survive the conditions of real life.

People do not try to preserve lean mass in a vacuum.

They try to do it while tired. While stressed. While under-slept. While rushed. While living inside days that keep narrowing their margin for good decisions.

Which means the next part of the obesity story is not really about motivation alone.

It is about recovery.

It is about exhaustion.

It is about the biology of a life that does not leave people well restored enough to live by what treatment recommends.

Chapter Seven: Sleep, Stress, and Time Poverty

The alarm goes off, but the night never really finished.

A child woke up. The phone lit up too late. The mind kept working after the body lay down. Morning arrives before recovery does. Coffee becomes breakfast or replaces it. Lunch gets pushed by meetings, traffic, patients, customers, emails, deadlines, or the ordinary disruptions that keep a modern day from staying inside its own lines. By late afternoon, the body is no longer making food decisions from a calm biological place. It is making them from accumulated sleep loss, background stress, and a shrinking amount of patience. Dinner now has to compete with exhaustion.

That scene is so ordinary that it often disappears into the background. We speak about obesity as if food choices were being made by fully restored people with time to plan, time to shop, time to cook, time to move, and time to sleep. Many choices are not made in that kind of life. They are made in tired lives.

This matters because obesity is not only a food story. It is also a recovery story.

Earlier in the book, I introduced a simple framework: calories influence body weight, macronutrient balance influences body composition, nutrient density influences health, and environment determines how hard or easy it is to live out the first three. Sleep, stress, and time pressure belong squarely in that fourth line. They shape what a person can sustain. They shape hunger, judgment, routine, and recovery. They shape whether the biology of good intentions ever gets a fair chance.

When people are under-slept, overextended, and chronically rushed, all four lines tend to drift in the wrong direction at once. It becomes easier to overconsume calories. It becomes harder to structure meals in a way that protects protein and muscle.

Diet quality erodes because convenience starts winning more decisions. And the environment becomes even more difficult to navigate because the person moving through it is now doing so in a depleted state.

Exhaustion is not a side issue in obesity.

It is part of the mechanism.

That truth is often missed because fatigue has been normalized. Many adults now live with such regular sleep debt, such regular strain, and such regular schedule pressure that they no longer experience those conditions as disruptions. They experience them as personality. Busy. Driven. Responsible. Needed. Productive. Behind. Pushing through. The body uses a different language. The body experiences those same conditions as stress load, shortened recovery, altered appetite, weaker impulse control, poorer glucose handling, and, over time, a greater tendency to live on whatever is fastest and easiest.

The body does not care whether the day looked respectable on a calendar. It still has to absorb the biology.

That is why this chapter matters. It is not an argument against hard work. It is not a complaint about ambition, discipline, caregiving, or responsibility. Work matters. Productivity matters. Family obligations matter. The point is more serious than that. Biological limits matter too. And when a culture repeatedly borrows from sleep, recovery, and time, the metabolic consequences should not surprise us.

A short night changes the next day long before dinner arrives.

Sleep is often treated like a luxury in modern life, as if it were mainly about comfort, mood, or personal preference. It is far more central than that. Sleep is biological maintenance. It is metabolic infrastructure. It is one of the conditions under which appetite, energy, hormone signaling, and judgment stay more stable.

When sleep is cut short, hunger often gets louder and fullness often gets quieter. A tired body is more likely to want quick comfort, quick reward, and quick energy. Foods high in sugar, refined starch, and fat often become more attractive, not because the person suddenly stopped caring about health, but because the brain under fatigue is drawn more strongly to what feels easy and rewarding. A short night can make calories look brighter and consequences look dimmer.

That is not weakness.

That is physiology under strain.

A tired brain also does not deliberate the same way a rested brain does. Self-regulation becomes more expensive. Planning becomes harder. Patience wears thin faster. Small choices start to feel larger than they should. A person may still know exactly what a healthier option looks like. Knowledge is not the problem. The problem is that the body making the choice is now working with less reserve.

This is one reason so much nutrition advice fails in practice. It assumes that knowing and doing exist in the same body at the same strength all day long. They do not. Many people know what they would like to eat at 8:00 a.m. The harder question is what feels realistic at 8:00 p.m., after a day has already used up most of their judgment.

Sleep loss affects more than appetite. It can also push the body toward poorer metabolic control in quieter ways. Blood sugar may be harder to regulate. Energy dips can feel sharper. Movement can feel less inviting. Strength training, which matters so much for preserving muscle during fat loss, can begin to feel optional in a life already running on fumes. Meal preparation, grocery planning, and even the effort of choosing better food can all weaken when the person is simply too tired to keep doing difficult things after dusk.

This is the hidden tax of poor sleep. It does not only make people feel bad. It makes healthy living cost more.

Some readers will already feel the other edge of this problem. Obesity can worsen sleep, and then poor sleep can worsen obesity in return. Excess adiposity can raise the risk of sleep apnea, a condition in which breathing repeatedly narrows or stops during sleep and sleep becomes fragmented even when the person spends enough hours in bed. So a person may be tired not only because life is crowded, but because sleep itself has been made less restorative. That creates a brutal loop. Poor sleep increases appetite and strain. Strain worsens metabolic health. Excess body fat worsens sleep further. The cycle can become self-reinforcing.

That loop is one reason obesity care should never treat sleep as an afterthought. A patient may be trying hard and still be attempting that work inside broken recovery.

No prescription can make five hours feel like eight.

Even the best treatment has to operate inside the body it is given.

Then there is stress.

Stress is one of those words that has become so common it risks sounding vague. But in real life, the experience is not vague at all. It is the body living with too many demands and too little relief. It is the nervous system staying activated longer than it was built to. It is the mind never fully standing down. It is financial pressure, caregiving pressure, work pressure, relationship strain, uncertainty, grief, noise, overload, and the steady mental labor of keeping a complicated life from coming apart.

Short bursts of stress are part of life. The body can handle challenge. It is built to respond. But chronic stress is different. Chronic stress is not a sprint. It is a background condition. The system never quite returns to baseline. The body keeps receiving the message that vigilance is still needed.

That has metabolic consequences.

A chronically stressed body often does not eat the same way a calm one does. Appetite can become more erratic. Cravings can become stronger. Highly rewarding foods can take on more pull. Not because the person is morally weak, but because food can become one of the fastest available forms of relief in a life that no longer offers many pauses. A sweet drink, a salty snack, a late-night dessert, a drive-through meal, something crunchy in the car, something easy while standing at the kitchen counter. These moments can look small. But under chronic strain, small moments are often where the physiology shows up.

The phrase stress eating can sound dismissive, almost playful, as if people are simply having a little extra comfort food after a hard day. The reality is often more serious. Stress eating is frequently an overloaded nervous system reaching for the fastest help it can find.

That is one reason shame is so unhelpful here. Shame misreads the event. It sees only the hand reaching for food. It does not see the accumulated strain behind the hand. It does not see the weeks of shortened sleep, the constant pressure, the decision overload, the absence of recovery, or the simple fact that many lives now offer almost no low-cost, rapidly available relief other than eating.

Food can become the most convenient form of relief in a hurried culture.

That does not make it harmless. It does make it understandable.

Stress also changes the texture of decision-making itself. A person under chronic strain becomes easier to wear down. This is where decision fatigue enters the picture. Most adults do not fail nutrition because they made one dramatic bad choice. They are more often defeated by the repeated cost of making many small good choices under pressure. Resist this. Plan that. Prepare this. Ignore that cue. Delay that urge. Stop there. Start over tomorrow. Repeat. Repeat. Repeat.

By evening, many people are not making a fresh decision. They are making the last decision of a depleted day.

That difference matters.

A well-rested, low-stress person with a stocked kitchen is taking one test. An under-slept, overbooked person with one eye on the clock and another on tomorrow's obligations is taking another. If those two people do not get the same result, we should be careful before turning the difference into a moral story.

Exhausted people do not live as if they are well-resourced people.

They do not shop the same way. They do not cook the same way. They do not snack the same way. They do not move the same way. They do not recover the same way. They do not make late-day decisions with the same reserve.

That is why time poverty belongs in the obesity conversation.

Time poverty is not just being busy. It is living with too little unclaimed time to carry out the basics of health with any consistency. It is not simply a full calendar. It is a life in which the margins have been stripped away. There is not enough flexible time to shop well, cook regularly, eat slowly, sleep adequately, move consistently, recover properly, and repeat the whole pattern tomorrow without strain.

Time poverty changes the meaning of food.

A food is not just calories, protein, or nutrient density. It is also the amount of life it asks for.

Does it require planning? Does it require a grocery run? Does it require chopping, cooking, and cleanup? Does it require a refrigerator that is stocked and a kitchen that is functioning? Does it require a predictable evening? Does it require energy that may already have been spent elsewhere?

These are not side questions. For many households, they are the real questions.

This is one reason convenience calories keep winning. They do not only deliver energy. They remove tasks. They reduce decisions. They save minutes. In a life that feels overscheduled, those features are not trivial. They are the point.

When people say they are too tired to cook, that sentence is often misunderstood. It can sound like an excuse to someone listening from a more buffered life. It is often a plain description of a real limit. Cooking is not only about willingness. It is about bandwidth. It is about whether there is still enough mind and body left to wash, chop, heat, time, plate, clean, and repeat while the rest of life keeps moving.

Healthy routines need margin.

That sentence deserves more respect than the culture usually gives it.

Meal planning needs margin. Protein-forward eating needs margin. Resistance training needs margin. Adequate sleep certainly needs margin. Even basic grocery maintenance needs margin.

Many people are living with very little of it.

Time poverty also pushes the day toward unnatural eating patterns. Breakfast gets skipped because the morning is compressed. Lunch is delayed because the meeting runs over, the shift stays busy, the classroom does not pause, the patients keep coming, the emails keep arriving, the work stack does not thin. By late afternoon or evening, the body has become both hungry and depleted. That combination is dangerous in a food environment full of easy reward. A person is now biologically ready to overcorrect and environmentally surrounded by foods that make overcorrection easy.

Then dinner arrives late.

Then portion control looks different.

Then nighttime eating becomes more likely, not because the person lacks principles, but because the body has been asked to make up too much ground too quickly.

This is one of the quiet links between time structure and obesity. A day with poor rhythm often produces a body with poor rhythm. Long gaps, rushed intake, convenience snacking, late heavy meals, eating while driving, eating while standing, eating while distracted, eating not from true hunger alone but from accumulated depletion. The body notices the disorder even when the calendar calls it normal.

Movement also becomes one of the first casualties of time scarcity. Not because exercise is unimportant, but because exercise usually competes poorly against deadlines, caregiving, commuting, and fatigue. Strength training, in particular, asks for a kind of intentionality that thin margins do not support well. Yet we already established in the last chapter that preserving muscle is essential during obesity treatment. So the life becomes even tighter. The patient is asked to eat better, preserve protein, protect sleep, and do resistance training while living in a schedule that barely leaves room for any of it.

This is where advice can begin to sound detached from reality.

A good recommendation delivered into a life with no margin can still fail.

That does not make the recommendation wrong. It means the structure around it is too weak.

One of the most overlooked ways people try to cope with time poverty is by borrowing from sleep. The day is crowded, so the only unclaimed time appears late at night. Some people stay up because they still have work to finish. Some because the house is finally quiet. Some because tomorrow is already coming and late night is the only hour that still feels partly theirs. The result is understandable and metabolically expensive. The person steals a little private time from sleep, then wakes under-recovered, and the whole cycle begins again with even less reserve than before.

This is how overworked lives become under-recovered bodies.

That sentence is not anti-work. It is pro-reality.

Hard work is honorable. Caregiving is honorable. Building a business, practicing medicine, driving long miles, teaching, serving, repairing, lifting, cleaning, studying, managing, and showing up for family are honorable forms of effort. The argument here is not against effort. The argument is against pretending that effort carries no biological cost when recovery is repeatedly removed.

Human beings can push hard. Human beings cannot push indefinitely without consequence.

A culture that celebrates endurance while neglecting restoration should not be surprised when metabolic health begins to fray.

This is especially true for people whose lives are organized around irregular or biologically difficult schedules. Shift work, night work, rotating schedules, unpredictable hours, and chronically interrupted sleep can create a deeper mismatch between the body's natural rhythms and the demands of income, service, and responsibility. Many essential workers live inside this mismatch for years. So do many clinicians. So do many parents. So do many people holding together more than one role at once.

Again, the answer is not condemnation. The answer is honesty.

If people are routinely asked to sleep at odd hours, eat at odd hours, work under artificial light, recover in fragments, and make nutritional decisions while fatigued, then weight regulation will often become harder. Blood sugar control may become harder. Structured eating may become harder. Consistency may become harder. The body is not being difficult. The body is responding to the pattern it is repeatedly given.

That has implications for treatment.

Serious obesity care cannot begin and end with a food list. It has to ask better questions about sleep, recovery, and schedule. How many hours is the person really sleeping? Is the sleep restorative or broken? Does the person snore, stop breathing, or wake unrefreshed? What time does the workday begin and end? How long is the commute? How unpredictable is the schedule? How much caregiving is happening after paid work ends? Where in the day does eating fall apart? When is hunger strongest? When does judgment get weakest? What is the real shape of fatigue in this life?

Without those questions, treatment remains too abstract.

A patient does not need a nutrition fantasy. A patient needs a fatigue-tested plan.

That might mean simplifying breakfast so the day does not begin in a metabolic hole. It might mean protecting some form of protein earlier in the day instead of asking dinner to repair everything later. It might mean using healthier convenience options strategically rather than pretending convenience itself can be abandoned. It might mean recognizing that the exhausted hour of the evening is where the plan is most likely to fail and building extra structure there. It might mean identifying and treating sleep apnea. It might mean adjusting expectations so that the plan fits the life that actually exists rather than the life the patient wishes they had.

A good clinician learns to ask where the day loses support.

That question is often more useful than asking where the person lacks motivation.

The answer might be 3:30 p.m., when the body crashes and the vending machine begins to look persuasive. It might be the commute home, when the car becomes a dining room. It might be 9:30 p.m., when food becomes a reward simply because the day finally stopped asking for something. It might be the early-morning rush, when breakfast disappears and the rest of the day inherits the damage.

When those break points become visible, the patient can be helped more respectfully and more realistically. Not with accusation, but with design.

This is also where the limits of downstream treatment come back into view. Medications may reduce appetite. They may help enormously. They deserve respect. But they do not create time. They do not shorten commutes. They do not protect bedtime. They do not automatically organize meals, repair a broken schedule, or give a strained household more margin. A medication can be powerful, but it still has to operate inside a life.

That is why upstream thinking matters so much. If sleep, stress, and time scarcity are part of the disease environment, then redesigning that environment becomes a legitimate health question. This does not require employers to become villains or work to become suspect. It requires a more mature view of human performance. Predictable schedules where possible, fewer avoidable disruptions, healthier food defaults, reasonable breaks, respect for sleep as a performance asset, and an honest willingness to see chronic fatigue as biologically consequential rather than merely inconvenient. None of that is anti-business. None of it is anti-discipline. It is pro-sustainability.

A high-performing society should care whether its people are living in a way their bodies can keep up with.

Productivity purchased by chronic under-recovery is often metabolic debt in disguise.

Medicine should be careful here, because not every overburdened life can be quickly redesigned. Some constraints are real. Income needs are real. Family needs are real. Many readers cannot simply decide to sleep more, work less, or create time that does not exist. That is exactly why blame is such a poor substitute for understanding. When a person is living with very little flexibility, the role of the clinician is not to moralize from a distance. It is to help create the strongest possible structure within the life that is actually being lived, while also being willing to say, honestly, that the structure around that person is part of the problem.

This is where compassion and seriousness have to stay together.

Compassion says: of course this is hard. Seriousness says: these conditions still matter biologically. Compassion says: you are not weak because tired life is harder to regulate. Seriousness says: if the tired life remains unchanged, the metabolic burden will often remain strong.

Good obesity medicine needs both voices.

There is another reason this chapter belongs where it does in the book. The last chapter argued that better treatment means losing fat while preserving muscle. But muscle preservation is not achieved by slogans. It requires protein, some intentional movement, and enough recovery for the body to respond well to the effort. A person who is chronically under-slept and chronically strained is being asked to protect lean mass from inside a physiologic environment that keeps nudging the other way. Recovery is not separate from body composition. It is one of the conditions that helps make body-composition improvement possible.

The same is true for diet quality. Nutrient-dense eating sounds simple until time scarcity enters the room. The same is true for the calorie line. Reasonable intake sounds obvious until hunger is made louder by short sleep and long stress. The same is true for the environmental line. The environment is not just food marketing and retail design. It is also schedule design, sleep opportunity, commute length, caregiving load, unpredictability, and whether the person has any room left in the day to live by what the clinic recommends.

The fourth line was never only about what sits on the shelf. It was also about what happens to a human being before that shelf is reached.

Once you see that, obesity looks less like a simple eating problem and more like what it often is: a condition shaped by chronic exposure, chronic convenience, and chronic under-recovery.

That does not erase agency. It explains the level of friction.

And it explains why so many people feel caught between what they know and what they can sustain. They are not only fighting appetite. They are fighting fatigue. They are not only choosing food. They are choosing under time pressure. They are not only trying to improve health. They are trying to do it while living inside schedules that keep draining the very capacities improvement requires.

This wider view also helps the culture ask better questions. Not only, What are people eating? But also, What kind of days are they living? How much sleep is the culture permitting? How much stress is the culture normalizing? How much ordinary time does the average household have for buying, preparing, and repeating a healthier pattern? What would it mean to design a society in which recovery was not treated as weakness and healthier routines did not require unusual heroism?

Those are not soft questions. They are structural ones.

And they lead us to an uncomfortable truth. Obesity is often discussed as though it begins when an adult finally gains too much weight. In reality, many of the pressures that shape appetite, routine, sleep, and food behavior begin far earlier than that. Children do not grow up outside the sleep patterns, stress patterns, and time pressures of the homes and institutions around them. They inherit the schedule before they inherit the diagnosis.

The rushed morning. The late dinner. The screen before bed. The fast food between activities. The snack used to quiet a hard evening. The family rhythm built around fatigue rather than restoration.

These are not merely adult problems that happen to occur in front of children. They are part of the childhood pipeline itself.

By the time a patient arrives in adulthood carrying obesity, the environment may have been training the biology for years.

You cannot fully understand obesity without understanding exhaustion.

And you cannot fully understand exhaustion without asking how early the schedule starts teaching it.

Chapter Eight: The Childhood Pipeline

A child is buckled into the back seat before the sun is fully up.

Breakfast is whatever can be carried in one hand, or it is postponed. School brings its own set of options. There may be a snack between classes, a rushed lunch, a classroom celebration, something from a vending area, something after practice, something on the ride home, and dinner at an hour when the day has already spent most of everybody's patience. Bedtime arrives late, and sleep begins under conditions that were not built for restoration.

None of this requires the child to understand calories, protein, nutrient density, appetite, or the long arc of metabolic health.

The environment understands first.

That is the argument of this chapter. Obesity is often discussed as though it begins when adult autonomy begins, as though the main story starts when a grown person is finally old enough to shop independently, order freely, drive to food, and be held fully responsible for every decision. But many metabolic stories begin much earlier than that. Long before adulthood, children are already learning what food is, what meals feel like, how often eating happens, what counts as normal sweetness, how big an ordinary portion looks, whether vegetables are expected or optional, whether water is ordinary or flavored calories are ordinary, whether dinner is seated or hurried, and whether sleep is protected or borrowed from the night.

Children do not inherit only genes.

They inherit menus, schedules, norms, and the emotional weather around food.

That matters because children are not small sovereign consumers. They do not set the household budget. They do not stock the pantry. They do not write school contracts. They do not choose what is placed at eye level near a register. They do not design sports leagues, lunch periods, advertising campaigns, or the timing of a family's evening. They eat inside decisions that adults and institutions have already made.

So when a society waits until adulthood to take obesity seriously, it has usually waited too long.

The phrase childhood pipeline is meant to make that visible. I do not use it to suggest that a child's future is fixed, or that early exposure creates some irreversible destiny. Pipelines can be interrupted. Paths can be changed. Children are not condemned by their environment forever. The point of seeing a pipeline is not to surrender to it. The point is to stop pretending the river starts at eighteen.

Many adult bodies arrive carrying childhood exposure.

That exposure begins with repetition. Children learn what is normal by living inside it again and again. What counts as breakfast. Whether snacks appear constantly or only occasionally. Whether meals have boundaries or whether eating drifts through the day. Whether fullness has time to speak before the next product opens. Whether food is mostly assembled from real ingredients or mostly torn open from packages. Whether the family rhythm makes room for sitting down or whether the day pushes everyone toward eating in motion.

Repetition is a teacher.

The body learns from it. Taste learns from it. Appetite learns from it. Expectation learns from it. What adults call preference is often partly memory. A child does not appear in the world already knowing that one level of sweetness feels ordinary and another feels extreme. A child learns what ordinary tastes like. A child learns what a meal is supposed to contain. A child learns whether protein is part of the structure, whether fruit and vegetables are familiar or rare, whether water belongs on the table, whether dessert is occasional or assumed, whether food solves boredom, whether food solves sadness, whether food arrives only at meals or trails through every compartment of the day.

This is one reason the first years matter so much. The palate is being taught. The daily script is being taught. The body is being introduced to its future defaults before it has any language to explain them.

And yet we should be careful here.

This is not a chapter written to frighten parents or recruit them into a new culture of dietary anxiety. Children do not need homes ruled by dietary fear. They do not need adults speaking about bodies with constant anxiety. They do not need every snack treated like a referendum on love or competence. The point is not perfection. The point is pattern.

A birthday cupcake is not the crisis.

A childhood built around constant reward food, constant grazing, weak meal boundaries, short sleep, and easy access to highly processed calories is different.

That difference is easy to miss because modern childhood has normalized so much of it. Pouches in the stroller. Crackers in the car seat. Bars in the backpack. Sweet drinks after games. Candy at checkout. A packaged snack handed over because the errand is still long, the line is still moving slowly, the child is still tired, the parent is still managing six things at once, and a small edible peace treaty seems cheaper than the conflict. None of these moments is proof of bad parenting. Most are proof of ordinary strain. But ordinary strain, repeated often enough, becomes a childhood environment.

That environment shapes the four-part model this book has returned to again and again. In childhood, just as in adulthood, calories influence body weight. Macronutrient balance influences body composition. Nutrient density influences health. And environment determines how hard or easy it is to live out the first three. The difference is that children have much less power over the fourth line.

Adults are still choosing around them.

Or more precisely, institutions are choosing around them, markets are choosing around them, schedules are choosing around them, and tired families are trying to survive inside those choices.

Genes matter, of course. Some children are biologically more vulnerable than others. Appetite differs. Satiety differs. The body's tendency to store energy differs. Hormones, medications, trauma, sleep disorders, developmental conditions, and family history all matter. But genes do not pack a lunchbox. Genes do not design a school menu. Genes do not place cartoon characters on a package. Genes do not decide whether a child sees food as a sit-down meal or as a constant background event. Biology may shape susceptibility. It does not erase exposure.

The childhood pipeline is built from both.

It is built from vulnerability and from what repeatedly lands on that vulnerability.

School is one of the places where this becomes most visible.

Children spend a large share of their waking hours in schools, child-care settings, and organized activities. That means these institutions do more than educate. They help teach what ordinary eating looks like. For many children, school meals are not a minor part of nutrition. They are an essential source of structure, stability, and nourishment. That has to be said clearly and respectfully. Many schools are doing difficult work under real constraints. Many children rely on those meals. Many school nutrition professionals are trying to serve health inside budgets, procurement rules, labor realities, student preferences, and time pressures that outsiders rarely see.

So the point here is not to attack schools.

The point is to recognize their power.

If a school day normalizes rushed lunches, frequent treats, low-satiety snacks, sweetened beverages, reward food, candy fundraisers, or classroom celebrations that repeatedly center sugar and ultra-processed food, then childhood metabolism is being shaped in public, not only at home. If lunch periods are short, children learn to eat fast. If the most visible and accepted foods are refined, convenient, and heavily packaged, children absorb that as ordinary. If physical activity is squeezed while food becomes ambient, the lesson is not delivered as ideology. It is delivered as routine.

Routine is persuasive.

One of the quiet features of modern childhood is how often food now appears outside traditional meals. A child may eat before school, in the classroom, at lunch, after school, at practice, at an event, in the car, during homework, and again late in the evening. The issue is not that children must never snack. The issue is that many children now grow up in a culture where eating has few natural stopping points. The body is not moving calmly from meal to meal. It is moving through a corridor of exposure.

That changes appetite. It changes expectation. It changes what hunger even feels like.

A child who is always within reach of some edible convenience may have fewer chances to experience the clear beginning of hunger and the clear ending of a meal. A child whose intake is built from frequent small processed foods may learn a very different relationship to fullness than a child who more often sits down to structured meals built around protein, fiber, and slower eating. Again, the issue is not one snack on one Tuesday. It is the architecture of ordinary life.

School and organized activities also shape the symbolic meaning of food. Pizza for achievement. Candy for good behavior. Donuts for celebration. Dessert as reward. A sweet treat because the day was hard. These customs are not malicious. They usually come from affection, community, or convenience. But they still teach. They teach children that food, especially highly rewarding food, is not only nourishment. It is also prize, relief, entertainment, and emotional punctuation.

By adolescence, the pipeline often widens.

Teenagers have more independence than younger children, but they are not yet fully free adults making decisions in a neutral marketplace. They are developing people inside a very aggressive commercial one. They begin carrying money, phones, social status concerns, and a deep need to belong. The food environment notices all of that quickly. So do advertisers.

Marketing to children and adolescents is not just about a commercial during a cartoon anymore. It is packaging, branding, celebrity influence, digital repetition, sports culture, social media, app-based ordering, convenience retail, gaming tie-ins, and the constant merging of food with identity. The goal is not merely to inform a young person that a product exists. The goal is to make the product feel normal, exciting, fun, adult, rebellious, comforting, social, or deserved.

Marketing does not simply sell food to children.

It helps script childhood around food.

That matters because children and adolescents are still learning what to trust, what to want, and what to imitate. Young children are especially impressionable. They do not interpret persuasion the way adults do. They respond to color, character, familiarity, repetition, and delight. Adolescents are more skeptical, but they are also navigating belonging, image, independence, and reward. They may know that they are being marketed to and still be strongly influenced by the association between food, social life, and self-definition.

A teenager walking out of school does not enter a philosophical debate about nutrient density.

That teenager enters a world of convenience stores, delivery apps, friends, after-school hunger, limited time, and products far more aggressively positioned than a piece of fruit or a protein-forward meal ever will be. If the culture keeps presenting sweet drinks, fried foods, oversized portions, and ultra-processed snacks as the easy language of freedom, fun, reward, or social belonging, then the metabolic consequences should not surprise us.

This is another reason obesity cannot be honestly described as an adult willpower story.

By the time willpower is being morally invoked, the child may already have spent years living in an environment organized against calm regulation.

At this point, many parents reading this may feel a tightening in the chest. That reaction deserves direct respect. Parents are already blamed for too much, and many mothers and fathers have spent years trying to do right by their children inside conditions they did not choose. Some are working long hours. Some are managing multiple jobs. Some are caring for elders in addition to children. Some are navigating food insecurity, neighborhood limits, school constraints, medical burdens, divorce, grief, or sheer exhaustion. Some are trying to stretch one paycheck across too many obligations. Some are simply doing the heroic, repetitive labor of family life without enough margin.

So let me say this plainly.

This is not an indictment of tired families.

It is an indictment of a system that keeps asking tired families to solve a systems problem one rushed evening at a time.

Parents are not trying to create a metabolically difficult childhood environment. Most are performing logistics under pressure. They are managing appetite, school pickup, homework, work messages, bedtime, budgets, sibling preferences, grocery gaps, traffic, sports, and the ordinary emotional weather of home. In that kind of life, convenience stops being a luxury and becomes a tool. A drive-through dinner can feel like rescue. A packaged snack can feel like insurance. A sweet food can feel like the fastest way to calm tears in a store aisle or survive one more late-afternoon transition. These are short-term solutions to real problems.

The system knows that. It makes products for exactly those moments.

This is where the last chapter on sleep, stress, and time poverty returns with even greater force. A child does not only eat the household diet. A child eats the household schedule. If the home runs late, the child runs late. If the adults are exhausted, the child often lives in that exhaustion too. If dinner happens after practice in the car, that becomes ordinary. If screens extend the evening because everybody still has tasks left, sleep gets thinner. If mornings are rushed, breakfast gets weaker or disappears. If weekends revolve around sports concessions, gas-station stops, and whatever can travel, that becomes part of the child's nutritional education.

Children inherit the family's time pressure before they ever understand the phrase.

They also absorb the family's emotional use of food. In a stressed household, food can become comfort, bargaining chip, distraction, peace offering, or reward. Again, that is not because parents are foolish. It is because food is fast. It is legal, available, portable, and usually more immediately effective than a deeper environmental fix that no one has time to implement on a Tuesday night.

The child learns that distress moves toward food. The child learns that celebration moves toward food. The child learns that boredom moves toward food. The child learns that a difficult evening can be softened with calories.

Those associations are human. Adults have them too. But when they are trained early and reinforced often, they become part of a long runway into later metabolic difficulty.

There is also a subtler issue that public conversation often misses. Children do not only learn what foods appear. They learn how food is organized. They learn whether meals have shape. They learn whether protein is part of the plate often enough to support fullness and growth. They learn whether fruit and vegetables are ordinary sights or occasional projects. They learn whether a beverage usually hydrates or usually sweetens. They learn whether eating happens with some attention or mostly while moving, scrolling, riding, or hurrying.

The form matters because the body notices more than flavor. A childhood built mostly from highly processed, low-fiber, low-protein convenience intake may not only shift body weight over time. It may also alter fullness, energy stability, body composition, and the child's sense of what eating is supposed to do. Food becomes something fast rather than something structured. Something constant rather than something bounded. Something rewarding first and nourishing second.

That is not a small lesson.

And by the time a child reaches adolescence, the body may already be fluent in it.

This is why prevention has to begin earlier than adult medicine usually begins speaking. If a nation waits for adulthood to address obesity, it is intervening after years of exposure have already done their work. The palate has been trained. The schedule has been trained. The family rhythm has been trained. The school rhythm has been experienced. The snack culture has been normalized. Sleep may already be thin. Shame may already have entered. A teenager may arrive in clinic feeling not only physically burdened but morally burdened, as though years of adult-designed exposure were somehow proof of personal failure.

That is a cruel misunderstanding.

It is also a strategic one.

Because prevention is not just earlier counseling. Prevention is earlier protection.

It means healthier defaults before disease-promoting patterns are deeply established. It means making the easier choice less metabolically destructive in the settings where children actually live. It means giving families more practical support, not more abstract blame. It means taking school food seriously enough to recognize that lunch trays and classroom norms are part of public health. It means noticing that sports culture, fundraising culture, convenience retail, and digital marketing are also part of the childhood food environment. It means treating sleep as pediatric infrastructure, not an optional lifestyle detail. It means helping parents preserve structure without demanding a level of time, money, and perfection that many do not have.

It also means understanding what prevention is not.

Prevention is not putting children on trial.

It is not teaching a ten-year-old to fear food. It is not turning childhood into a calorie-counting project. It is not making a child feel watched, appraised, or cosmetically judged. It is not producing a new generation of young people whose bodies look smaller while their relationship with food becomes anxious.

That would not be wisdom. That would be another kind of harm.

The goal is not to raise smaller children at any cost. The goal is to raise well-supported children. Better-fed children. Better-rested children. Children whose lives contain more structure, more real nourishment, more chances for regular meals, more protection from constant marketing, and fewer situations in which highly processed convenience food becomes the default answer to every strain.

In other words, the aim is health, not fear.

That distinction matters because public discussion around childhood weight can become morally clumsy very quickly. Some people grow so afraid of stigma that they stop speaking clearly about disease risk. Others grow so anxious about disease that they begin speaking about children and bodies in ways that are harsh, humiliating, or obsessive. Both responses fail.

A child living with obesity is not a cautionary symbol for adults to discuss at a distance. That child is a child. That child deserves dignity, medical seriousness, emotional safety, and relief from lazy judgment. But dignity does not require us to pretend the physiology is irrelevant. The body does not wait until adulthood to respond to prolonged exposure. Complications can begin early. Sleep can worsen early. Mobility can become harder early. The burden can become real long before the culture feels comfortable naming it.

That is one reason early prevention matters so much. The earlier we protect the environment, the less often we force children into the impossible position of absorbing both the disease burden and the stigma around the disease. A society that leaves the pipeline intact is not neutral. It is just intervening late and blaming early.

Better prevention would ask different questions.

Not only, "What should this child weigh?" But also, "What is the child's food environment?" "What does the school day feed?" "What does the household schedule permit?" "How much sleep is this child actually getting?" "Where does the day fall apart?" "What foods are easy in this neighborhood, this budget, this routine?" "What kind of marketing is surrounding this child?" "What kind of support does this family actually have?"

Those are more serious questions than the scale alone can answer. They are also kinder questions, because they look for structure instead of immediately searching for fault.

The physician's role will become more explicitly upstream later in this book. For now, it is enough to say that childhood prevention should not live only in slogans about personal responsibility delivered after patterns are already established. It should live in earlier access, earlier structure, earlier protection, and earlier honesty about the environments in which children are being raised.

It should also make us humbler about adult obesity treatment.

When an adult walks into clinic with obesity, that adult may not be starting at zero. The body standing in front of us may carry years of childhood normalization behind it: years of sweet drinks seen as ordinary, years of school and activity food organized around convenience, years of rushed dinners, reward snacks, short sleep, emotional eating cues, and constant exposure to highly processed products. Adult medicine is then trying to reverse a pattern that may have been rehearsed for a very long time.

That does not make treatment hopeless.

But it should make treatment more compassionate. And it should make prevention more urgent.

The childhood pipeline also helps explain why the public conversation so often goes wrong. People look at adult obesity and imagine a series of isolated adult decisions. They see the final visible stage and miss the earlier invisible training. They see the body at forty and forget the pantry at eight, the lunch line at ten, the sports drinks at twelve, the late dinners at thirteen, the social marketing at fifteen, the short sleep all along the way. They see the endpoint and invent a moral story about the person. Meanwhile, the environment has been tutoring the pattern for years.

Once you see that, the old language starts to sound thinner than it did before.

“Why doesn’t this person make better choices?” Compared with what early defaults? Inside what learned normal? Against what repeated cues? With what history of family strain, school exposure, short sleep, food reward, and commercial persuasion already in place?

These questions do not erase responsibility. They enlarge explanation. And serious medicine needs enlarged explanation if it wants better outcomes than blame has produced.

The larger lesson is simple, even if the implications are not.

Obesity is often a pipeline problem, not just an adult decision problem.

That means the work cannot begin only in the adult clinic. It cannot begin only after blood sugar rises, sleep worsens, liver fat accumulates, or shame has already entered the picture. It cannot begin only after the body has spent years living inside patterns it did not design. If we want fewer adults burdened by obesity, we have to become more serious about the environments training children long before adult autonomy arrives.

That will require more than nutrition slogans. It will require a wider lens: family schedules, school food, advertising, snack norms, sleep protection, practical support for parents, and a more honest account of what modern childhood has become. It will require remembering that children do not merely grow inside bodies. They grow inside systems.

And systems teach early.

That truth should change both our urgency and our tone. It should make us move earlier. It should also make us gentler with the people already living in the result. By the time many children become adolescents, and many adolescents become adults, blame is already badly misdirected. But denial is not the answer either. If we are going to care well for people, we need a moral language strong enough to reject shame without retreating from truth.

Once we see how early the pipeline begins, one thing becomes harder to defend: stigma.

Another thing becomes harder to defend too: the comforting fiction that common disease is not really disease.

We need a way to protect dignity without softening the truth.

That is where we turn next.

Chapter Nine: Dignity Without Denial

Before the first question is asked, the apology arrives.

A person steps onto a clinic scale, sits down on the exam table, and begins trying to explain before any real medicine has started. The body has already been placed on trial. The visit is supposed to be about health, but the room is crowded with something older and harsher than health. It is crowded with judgment.

That scene matters because obesity lives inside one of the most confused moral conversations in modern medicine.

It is a real disease, with real metabolic and functional consequences. It is also one of the most stigmatized conditions in public life. So the culture keeps lurching between two failures. One failure tells people they should feel ashamed. The other, reacting against that cruelty, becomes afraid to say clearly that there is a real medical problem to name.

Neither response serves patients.

This chapter is about refusing both.

The way through begins with a distinction the culture keeps losing. Human worth and metabolic health are not the same category. Worth is unconditional. Health is biological. Worth does not rise and fall with a lab result, a waist measurement, or a number on a scale. Health can improve or worsen. Disease can be present or absent. A person can be fully worthy and still need treatment.

That should not be a radical sentence. In a healthier culture, it would be obvious.

We do not make people audition for dignity when their blood pressure rises. We do not tell them they are more deserving of respect if their cholesterol improves. We do not withhold courtesy until the A1c is lower. Yet obesity has too often been treated as an exception, as though body size were not merely a health topic but a moral referendum.

That is where stigma enters.

Stigma is not only mockery. It is not only the joke, the stare, the casual insult, or the internet cruelty that turns another person's body into public entertainment. It is also the quieter assumption that a larger body must reflect laziness, ignorance, weak character, or poor self-control. It is the belief that someone's size can tell you something final about their discipline, intelligence, seriousness, or worth.

It cannot.

If you have ever delayed an appointment because you did not want to be weighed, lectured, or looked at with disappointment, then you already know that stigma is not an abstract problem. It changes behavior. It teaches people to protect themselves from care before they can receive care. It makes the clinic feel less like refuge and more like exposure.

That is one reason shame is such a poor strategy in obesity medicine.

Shame does not improve metabolic health. It does not lower blood sugar by itself. It does not strengthen sleep, improve body composition, or make the modern food environment less aggressive. What it often does is drive silence, self-blame, avoidance, and desperate short-term efforts that leave people more exhausted than before.

Some people have been taught to think that disgust is a useful source of motivation. If they feel bad enough, perhaps they will finally change. If they are embarrassed enough, perhaps they will become disciplined. If they are frightened enough by their own reflection, perhaps they will do what health requires.

That is one of the crueler myths in modern health.

Self-contempt is brittle fuel. It may produce bursts of punishment. It rarely produces durable care.

No one should have to hate their body in order to help it.

That sentence matters more than it may first appear. A great deal of weight-related suffering is worsened not only by the biology of disease, but by the belief that care must begin with contempt. Many people have spent years trying to become harsh enough with themselves to finally improve. They assume kindness will make them complacent. They assume softness toward themselves will remove the last source of pressure.

In practice, the opposite is often closer to the truth. A person who feels constantly accused becomes harder to help, not easier. A person who feels reduced to a body size has less reason to trust the conversation. A person who has been humiliated enough times may stop seeking help altogether.

The cruelest version of stigma is the one that moves indoors.

After enough public judgment, people often begin speaking to themselves in a voice no clinician should ever use. Every struggle becomes evidence against their character. Every setback becomes proof that they are uniquely broken. The entire history of processed food, cheap calories, sleep loss, chronic stress, time scarcity, genetics, medication effects, childhood exposure, family patterns, and metabolic vulnerability gets collapsed into one punishing story: I should have been able to control this.

But that story is too small.

This book has spent several chapters widening the frame. The country did not suddenly lose willpower. The food environment changed. Cheap calories became easier to live on. Sleep grew thinner. Stress became ordinary. Childhood exposure began earlier. Better treatment requires attention to body composition, muscle, function, and recovery, not just to pounds. Once those realities are visible, shame starts looking not only cruel, but badly outdated.

It is not medicine. It is misdiagnosis wearing a moral tone.

Stigma also has a distinctly clinical form, and it is often less theatrical than the public kind. In medicine, stigma frequently appears as reductionism. The patient disappears behind the weight. Every complaint is filtered through one crude assumption. Knee pain is presumed before it is examined. Fatigue is attributed before sleep is discussed. Shortness of breath is simplified before a fuller evaluation is done. The larger patient receives a reflex instead of a workup.

That is not precision.

It is laziness.

A person living with obesity deserves the same seriousness any other patient deserves. That means a real history. A real differential diagnosis. Real curiosity. Real equipment that fits. Real seating. Real gowns. Real blood pressure cuffs. A room that communicates belonging rather than embarrassment. These are not cosmetic details of care. They are part of the architecture of dignity.

Respect should be ordinary in medicine. It should not have to be earned.

And yet another problem appears the moment we say all of this clearly. Because the cruelty is real, many people have understandably become suspicious of any conversation about obesity that sounds moralized, aesthetic, or simplistic. They know the scale is crude. They know thinness and virtue are not the same thing. They know a person can live in a larger body and still be intelligent, active, loving, competent, generous, and fully deserving of admiration. They know that body size has been used to humiliate children, dismiss adults, and distort clinical conversations.

All of that is true.

But a true correction can still overshoot.

In trying to protect people from stigma, the culture is sometimes tempted toward a different error. It begins to speak as though obesity is only a social judgment, or only a cosmetic label, or only a problem of prejudice. It becomes so uncomfortable with the history of shame that it hesitates to say plainly that excess and dysregulated body fat can impose real burden on the body.

This, too, fails patients.

The opposite of stigma is not denial. It is dignity.

Dignity says that every person deserves respect, belonging, and humane care regardless of body size. Denial says that because respect is nonnegotiable, obesity itself must not be discussed as a disease when it is functioning as one. Those are not the same claim. They should never be confused.

A body can deserve unconditional respect and still be under real metabolic strain.

That distinction is not a technicality. It is the whole chapter.

When the culture loses it, the conversation becomes muddy very quickly. A reader may hear that weight does not equal worth, which is true, and from there slide into the idea that body fat therefore has no ordinary physiologic consequences, which is false. Or a clinician may know that BMI is incomplete, which is true, and from there become reluctant to discuss obesity at all, which is not careful medicine. Or a public discussion may recoil so hard from body-shaming that it begins treating obesity as though it were merely a beauty debate in disguise.

It is not.

Obesity is not a beauty standard. It is not a fashion disagreement. It is not just about appearance.

The issue is not that a larger body offends someone's aesthetic preference. The issue is that excess and dysregulated body fat can change blood sugar, burden the liver, raise the risk of sleep apnea, worsen blood pressure, stress joints, reduce stamina, and make the body harder to live in over time. The burden may be metabolic. It may be mechanical. It may be functional. Often it is several things at once.

That is why the last several chapters insisted on more precision. Weight is not the same as health. Weight is not the same as body composition. BMI is not the whole story. Some people at lower weights are metabolically unwell. Some people at higher weights do not fit the crude stereotype the culture expects. Fat distribution matters. Muscle matters. Function matters. A number alone does not tell the whole clinical story.

But greater precision should make us more honest, not less.

The fact that weight is an incomplete measure does not mean adiposity is irrelevant. The fact that the scale is crude does not mean disease disappears. The fact that stigma exists does not mean the physiology becomes optional.

A disease does not stop being a disease because the topic became politically uncomfortable.

This matters because false reassurance can wound people too.

There is a kind of softness that comforts the moment and fails the future. It tells a person, directly or indirectly, that the main problem is other people's judgment, while the body is quietly sending other signals: worsening snoring, more fatigue, rising blood sugar, aching knees, climbing breathlessness, a liver storing fat, a body carrying more mechanical and metabolic burden than it should.

Social cruelty can be real.

Metabolic strain can be real at the same time.

Patients should not be forced to choose which truth they are allowed to speak.

This is one reason obesity should never be treated as merely cosmetic. Cosmetic concerns belong mostly to appearance. Obesity, when present as disease, belongs to the deeper category of biology and function. It changes what the body is carrying and how the body is coping. It can shape sleep, movement, liver health, insulin resistance, blood pressure, fertility, pain, mobility, and long-term disease risk. It can narrow the margin of daily life.

A person may first notice this not through a diagnosis, but through small losses. Stairs feel steeper. The body feels heavier by late afternoon. The seat belt shortens. The shoes become harder to tie. Sleep becomes noisier. Clothing becomes only the visible part of a much larger experience. The issue is not vanity. The issue is that daily life may be becoming more burdened from the inside and the outside at the same time.

The culture often gets this backward. It assumes obesity matters because it is visible.

Often it matters more because of what is less visible.

That is one reason medications and surgery deserve respect rather than ridicule. People do not seek serious obesity treatment because a mirror disappointed them one morning and they have no deeper concerns. They seek treatment because the burden is real. Because the body is harder to carry. Because blood sugar is rising. Because the liver is changing. Because sleep is breaking. Because previous attempts have failed. Because the disease is doing what disease does.

When that burden is real, calling it real is not cruelty.

It is accuracy.

And accuracy, handled correctly, can be merciful.

That may sound counterintuitive in a culture that has so often used health language as a mask for contempt. But many people feel a deep relief when medicine finally stops speaking in moral code and starts speaking plainly. The conversation changes. It moves from What is wrong with me as a person to What is happening in my body, and what can we do about it?

That change matters.

A diagnosis should name a burden, not assign a blame.

At its best, disease language can actually lower shame rather than deepen it, because it puts the struggle back into the category of the understandable and the treatable. It says this is not merely a private failure of character. There is biology here. There is environment here. There is physiology, exposure, habit, sleep, stress, muscle, appetite, childhood patterning, food design, and modern commercial pressure here. There is a real clinical story here.

Truth can be merciful because it gives the suffering a context larger than self-contempt.

It can also be merciful because it permits seriousness. A disease that cannot be named clearly often cannot be treated clearly. If obesity is softened into a topic of appearance alone, it becomes easier for institutions to trivialize it, easier for health systems to underinvest in it, easier for employers and schools to ignore upstream contributors, easier for policymakers to treat it as private failure, and easier for families to keep suffering without a stronger language for what is happening.

There is a kind of politeness that is really abandonment.

A clinician who sees clear metabolic burden and stays silent out of discomfort may feel gentle in the moment. But if the silence leaves the patient alone with worsening sleep apnea, worsening fatty liver, worsening blood sugar, or worsening function, it is not the full kind of care the patient deserves. Silence can feel kind in the room and careless over time.

That does not mean every conversation about body size must begin with the word obesity, or with a lecture, or with a scale-centered script. Good care is more skillful than that. It asks permission. It listens first. It focuses on health, function, symptoms, sleep, goals, and lived barriers. It uses respectful language. It notices what the patient has already carried. It remembers that the person in front of you may have tried many times and may already be expecting dismissal.

Good care sounds like partnership, not prosecution.

It also refuses another common error: using weight as an automatic explanation for everything. A patient in a larger body deserves more than a reflex. If there is pain, investigate pain. If there is fatigue, investigate fatigue. If there is shortness of breath, investigate shortness of breath. Obesity may be part of the story. It is not permission to stop thinking.

Respect requires seriousness in both directions. Serious enough to treat obesity when it is clinically present. Serious enough not to let obesity replace good medicine.

This steadier middle path is harder than either extreme. Stigma is easy because it simplifies the world into blame. Denial is easy because it avoids discomfort. Dignity without denial requires something better. It requires separating categories the culture keeps fusing together.

Worth is one category. Health is another.

A person's worth is not improved by lower body fat. A person's worth is not diminished by higher body fat. Health, however, can improve or worsen depending on what the body is carrying and what that tissue is doing.

Once those categories are separated, much of the confusion begins to clear.

You can reject weight-based contempt without pretending disease is harmless. You can speak honestly about obesity without reducing a person to it. You can respect every body in public life without declaring every metabolic state equally benign. You can make room for belonging without asking biology to lie.

This is the difference between respecting people and normalizing disease.

Respecting people means they deserve competent care, humane design, ordinary courtesy, fair treatment, and social belonging at every body size. It means a child should not be mocked. It means that a person's body is not public territory. No one forfeits privacy, dignity, or basic respect because their weight is visible. It means a patient should not be shamed into silence. It means a clinic, school, workplace, and public setting should not turn body size into humiliation.

Normalizing disease is something else. It means allowing widespread metabolic harm to become invisible simply because it is now common. It means mistaking prevalence for safety. It means deciding that because a condition affects many people, calling it a condition must somehow be offensive. It means letting the body's burden disappear into the culture's discomfort.

That is not compassion.

That is drift.

Common is not the same as healthy. Familiar is not the same as harmless. A society can become used to larger portions, poorer sleep, lower fitness, rising fatty liver, worsening blood sugar, more adolescent prediabetes, more sleep apnea, more chronic fatigue, and more bodies living under metabolic strain. But habituation is not the same as health. It is just adaptation of the eye.

The body does not care that the eye has adapted.

This is especially important because the current food and work environment benefits when the public conversation gets trapped in the wrong argument. Stigma blames the person. Denial blurs the diagnosis. Both leave the deeper system largely untouched. The cheap-calorie economy remains intact. The sleep debt remains intact. The childhood pipeline remains intact. The school and retail defaults remain intact. The patient gets blamed or vaguely reassured, and the upstream machinery keeps running.

In that sense, the false choice between shame and denial is convenient for the system.

It is not convenient for the patient.

A culture can make disease-promoting defaults ordinary upstream and then shame people downstream. That may be one of the ugliest features of the modern obesity story. The same world that saturates daily life with cheap, easy, engineered calories can then turn around and moralize the bodies shaped by that exposure. Or, when the cruelty becomes impossible to ignore, the culture can swing toward a softer error and act as though the burden is not really burden at all.

Both approaches hide the same larger failure.

Neither asks enough of institutions. Neither redesigns the environment. Neither gives the patient the truer map.

The truer map says this: people deserve dignity at every size, and obesity can still be disease when it is clinically present. Those statements do not fight each other. They complete each other.

That is also why the phrase body positivity, or body acceptance, helps some people and confuses others. The helpful part is morally important. No one should have to earn love, visibility, or belonging by shrinking. No one should have to begin health by hating themselves. No child should be taught that their body is an embarrassment. No adult should be told that they must become more acceptable before they become fully human in the public eye.

All of that deserves a strong yes.

But if acceptance drifts into the suggestion that obesity itself carries no meaningful medical risk, then the medicine gets blurry. A body can be accepted socially and still need treatment clinically. Belonging and biology are not enemies. They live in different categories.

Belonging should not depend on body size. Treatment should begin with dignity, not shame.

That is the balance.

The same is true for the way physicians lead the public conversation. Medicine should not borrow the language of disgust from the culture. It should not use humiliation as motivation. It should not confuse concern with scolding. But it should also not become so nervous about offense that it stops naming real disease or advocating for real prevention.

Physicians are trained, at our best, to tell the truth without moralizing it. We do this with high blood pressure, heart failure, sleep apnea, asthma, depression, cancer, kidney disease, and dozens of other burdens that can change a life without changing a person's worth. Obesity deserves that same steadiness. Not panic. Not cruelty. Not euphemism so vague it cannot support a plan. Plain truth, respectful language, and real help.

That steadiness should shape public health too. Campaigns built on humiliation are morally cheap and strategically weak. They may get attention. They rarely build trust. But public health that becomes so soft it cannot say processed food, body fat distribution, sleep, and metabolic disease are real problems is weak in a different way. One version wounds people by contempt. The other leaves them underinformed while the burden grows.

A humane culture should reject both.

It should say, without hesitation, that mockery is unacceptable. It should also say, without hesitation, that obesity is not merely cosmetic when it is burdening health.

It should say that every person deserves decent treatment now. It should also say that the nation should want less disease tomorrow.

It should widen furniture, language, design, and belonging for the bodies people are living in now. It should also widen access to better food, better sleep, better recovery, and better prevention so fewer people are pushed toward disease later.

Those are not competing moral visions. They are two obligations of the same serious society.

There is another kind of mercy in truth, and it may be the most important one. When obesity is named honestly and respectfully, it becomes easier to move from blame to strategy. The question stops being Why can't you control yourself? and becomes What forces are acting on this body, what burden is already present, and what support will actually help? That is a much better question. It is clinically better. It is also morally cleaner.

It makes room for history. It makes room for genetics. It makes room for medication effects, injuries, trauma, depression, sleep loss, shift work, time scarcity, food access, family stress, childhood patterning, and the cheap-calorie environment we have already traced through this book. It makes room for biology without erasing agency. It makes room for agency without assigning all of the blame to the individual.

That is what a truer map does. It lowers accusation and raises understanding. It does not excuse disease. It explains disease well enough to treat it seriously.

This is the chapter's central tension, but it is also its resolution. We do not have to choose between kindness and clarity. The choice was false from the beginning.

Compassion without honesty becomes sentiment. Honesty without compassion becomes contempt. People living with obesity deserve neither false reassurance nor humiliation. They deserve medicine serious enough to tell the truth and humane enough to leave shame out of it.

They deserve to hear that body size is not a moral score. They deserve to hear that health is not identical to appearance. They deserve to hear that obesity is not the same thing as personal failure. They deserve to hear that when excess adiposity is burdening health, that burden is real. They deserve to hear that treatment can help. They deserve to hear that systems matter.

They deserve to hear that their worth does not depend on the outcome.

Most of all, they deserve not to be stranded between two bad stories. One says you are the problem. The other says there is no problem. The truth is harder, kinder, and far more useful.

The problem is not the worth of the person. The problem is the burden on the body. And the body lives inside systems that often make the burden harder to avoid and harder to treat.

Once that becomes clear, another failure in the national response becomes impossible to ignore. If obesity is a real disease and shame does not help, then a brief lecture was never going to be enough. If the environment is strong and the burden is real, then advice without structure was always too weak. If patients deserve more than blame and more than denial, they also deserve more than slogans.

That is where we turn next.

Chapter Ten: Why Advice Alone Fails

The visit ends with familiar instructions.

Eat less. Move more. Cut back on sugar. Watch the portions. Try to exercise. Get serious about your health.

None of that is false. Most of it is directionally true. And yet many patients leave appointments like that with a quiet feeling that something important has been missed.

It has.

Because between a true sentence and a lived life, there is a long distance.

By the time the patient reaches the parking lot, the advice is already competing with the rest of the day. The commute is still there. The work schedule is still there. The under-slept night is still there. The pantry is still there. The break room is still there. The drive-through lights are still there. The children still need dinner. The grocery bill still matters. The hour of low judgment at the end of the day is still waiting.

Nothing in the environment has changed. Only the instructions have.

This chapter is not an argument against lifestyle change. It is an argument against underpowered lifestyle treatment.

Lifestyle matters deeply in obesity medicine. Food matters. Sleep matters. Movement matters. Muscle matters. Recovery matters. Daily structure matters. They matter so much, in fact, that it is not enough to mention them briefly and call the job done. A chronic disease shaped by a powerful environment deserves more than a few correct sentences.

That is where the modern conversation keeps getting stuck. Many people hear a criticism of simplistic advice and assume the criticism must be that the advice itself is wrong. That is not the point. The point is that telling people what matters is not the same as helping them build a life around it.

Advice is not the same thing as treatment.

It can be part of treatment. Sometimes it is an important part. But if obesity is a serious chronic disease, and if the modern environment is repeatedly pushing in the wrong direction, then handing a person brief instructions and expecting durable change was never a serious national strategy.

That is one reason so many patients have walked away from care feeling not only disappointed, but blamed. The advice sounds simple. The execution is not. When the simple message fails, the patient often assumes the failure must belong to them.

But often the deeper truth is harder and kinder than that.

The advice was too small for the setting in which it had to survive.

That becomes easier to see once we name a reality that much of public health still avoids. Most adults do not lack basic information about food. They may be confused on the margins. They may disagree about details. They may not know the answer to every nutritional argument passing across the internet. But most already know the broad outlines.

They know sugary drinks are not helping them.

They know vegetables are not the problem.

They know that eating in the car most nights is probably not an ideal long-term plan.

They know sleep matters, even if they do not have enough of it.

They know that fast food, vending food, gas-station food, and highly processed snack food are different from a well-structured meal.

The knowledge is often already there.

What is usually missing is not information alone. What is missing is feasible repetition.

That distinction matters because obesity is not mostly a problem of knowing once. It is a problem of doing repeatedly. The real question is not whether a person can correctly answer a nutrition quiz in a clinic waiting room. The real question is whether the pattern can survive Monday morning, a stressful Wednesday, a late Thursday, a weekend of errands, a family birthday, a poor night of sleep, an overbooked workday, and the familiar tired hour when dinner still has to happen and the easiest calories are the ones already waiting.

Knowing what to do is important.

Being able to do it, again and again, inside a pressured life is the harder problem.

This is where the old phrase eat less and move more begins to show its weakness.

It is not wrong. It is unfinished.

It is directionally true in the way spend less and save more is directionally true. Anyone can say it. It points in the general direction of the goal. But it does not tell a real person how to live there. It does not tell them what breakfast will happen when the morning is compressed. It does not tell them how to handle the 3:30 p.m. crash and the vending machine. It does not tell them how to protect protein so the body does not lose too much muscle along with fat. It does not tell them how to build movement into a life already short on time. It does not tell them what to do on the night when the refrigerator is thin and the family is hungry and the house does not contain much moral drama left to spend.

A slogan can point.

A structure has to carry.

That is why brief advice so often fails at scale. It names the destination while leaving the road mostly undesigned.

And yet human behavior is exquisitely sensitive to design.

People eat what is visible, what is easy, what is affordable, what is acceptable to the household, what is already in the car, what can be prepared without much thought, what promises quick relief, and what fits the time and energy still available. They do not do this because they are uniquely weak. They do it because human beings, like human beings always have, respond to convenience, fatigue, reward, routine, and friction.

If a healthier choice requires planning, shopping, chopping, cooking, cleanup, resistance from family members, and more patience than the hour contains, while the less healthy choice requires only a short drive and a card swipe, then the two choices are not competing on equal terms.

If a person is told to move more, but the instruction remains vague, the workday remains packed, the commute remains long, and the body remains under-recovered, then the plan is not really a plan yet. It is a wish wearing the clothes of advice.

The same is true for eating less. Eat less what? In what structure? With what replacement? While preserving protein? While staying full enough to function? While living amid constant exposure to cheap, easy calories? While protecting enough strength and muscle to avoid becoming a smaller, weaker version of yourself? A command that ignores those questions is not a mature clinical intervention.

The distance between knowing and doing is where obesity medicine either becomes real or stays rhetorical.

To become real, behavior change has to be much more concrete than the public conversation usually allows. It has to move from general virtue language into daily architecture.

What time is breakfast, and what will it actually be?

Where will protein come from early in the day?

What will happen during the late-afternoon hunger window?

What is the emergency dinner for the night that falls apart?

Which foods in the home are most likely to defeat the person's best intentions when fatigue rises?

What is the plan for beverages?

What movement is realistic this week, not in fantasy, but in the calendar as it actually exists?

How will sleep be protected, or if it cannot be fully protected, how will the eating plan become more defensive on tired days?

Where does the plan usually fail the patient?

That last question is often more useful than which diet is best.

A good obesity clinician learns to ask where the day breaks.

For one person, the day breaks at breakfast because the morning is too rushed and the first real intake comes as sugary coffee and whatever can be grabbed on the way to work. For another, it breaks at midafternoon because hunger and fatigue arrive at the same moment and the easiest available food is highly processed. For another, it breaks on the commute home because the body is hungry, dinner is distant, and the car passes fifteen convenient sources of quick reward before reaching the front door. For another, it breaks after dinner, when the children are finally down, the house is quiet, and eating becomes the fastest remaining form of relief.

Those break points matter because sustained behavior change is usually not built by trying to be perfect everywhere. It is more often built by getting strategic at the points where the pattern repeatedly fails.

That kind of support looks less glamorous than the culture's transformation stories. It is not mostly about inspiration. It is about precision. It is about designing around predictable weakness rather than pretending predictable weakness should not exist.

If afternoon hunger predictably knocks the day off course, then a structured lunch, adequate protein, and a planned bridging option may matter more than one more lecture about personal responsibility.

If late-night eating repeatedly follows short sleep and emotional depletion, then sleep protection and evening structure may matter more than generic advice about portion control.

If the household runs on convenience because the week leaves no margin for elaborate cooking, then healthier convenience becomes part of the answer. Frozen vegetables. Rotisserie chicken. Plain Greek yogurt. Pre-washed greens. Higher-protein staples. Ready beans. Cut fruit. Soup that can actually become dinner. Emergency food that makes the next best choice possible when the night falls apart.

The best plan is usually not the purest one.

It is the one robust enough to survive real life.

That is one of the great missed truths in obesity care. A plan that works only when the patient is rested, home early, highly motivated, and shopping in a well-stocked store on a calm Sunday afternoon is not a serious treatment plan. A serious treatment plan has to survive Thursday at 7:15 p.m.

This is also why sustained behavior change requires repetition and follow-up.

A single educational visit cannot carry what daily pressure keeps unloading. The patient sees the clinic a handful of times a year. The environment makes contact several times before lunch. The grocery store repeats itself. The workweek repeats itself. The family rhythm repeats itself. Appetite repeats itself. Fatigue repeats itself. Exposure repeats itself.

Effective care has to repeat too.

Not because people are childish. Because people are human.

Habits are not learned once and then stored in perfect condition. They are strengthened or weakened by repetition, context, mood, convenience, household patterns, and stress. A better eating structure may work for three days, then run into travel, conflict, illness, money pressure, or poor sleep. Without follow-up, the person is left alone with the setback and tends to interpret it as proof of failure. With follow-up, the setback can be read more honestly, as information.

This is what meaningful support does. It turns rough weeks into data instead of verdicts.

Where did the plan fail?

What part was too fragile?

What hour is still unprotected?

What food is still too available?

What hunger signal is still too strong?

What piece of the household routine needs to be reworked?

When treatment is built this way, the tone changes. The patient is no longer being judged from a distance. The patient is being helped through a real problem.

That is closer to how medicine is supposed to feel.

It is also closer to how other chronic diseases are treated. We do not usually tell a patient with poorly controlled high blood pressure to care more, reduce the salt, exercise more, and then vanish into the year. We follow up. We reassess. We intensify. We add tools. We interpret imperfect control as a sign that the treatment plan needs more strength, not as proof that the patient is undeserving of care.

Obesity deserves that same seriousness.

But obesity has long been treated differently because it has long been moralized differently. As long as the culture sees excess weight as a simple referendum on character, it will keep confusing education with treatment. It will act as though a few reminders should be enough if the patient cares deeply enough. And when they are not enough, it will quietly assign the gap to personal failure rather than to the mismatch between a strong disease environment and a weak intervention.

That is one of the moral injuries built into obesity care.

Patients are often asked to interpret a structurally predictable failure as a private flaw.

A person hears simple advice. The person cannot sustain it. The person does not conclude that ultra-processed food, long work hours, chronic fatigue, household strain, constant cue exposure, and underpowered clinical support were too much for a pamphlet to overcome. The person concludes that they must be lazy, weak, unserious, broken, or beyond help.

The system speaks in short instructions.

The patient absorbs the blame in long form.

Anyone who has spent time in obesity care has seen what that does. It makes people apologize before they are examined. It makes them delay appointments. It makes them try cycles of overrestriction that cannot last. It makes them hide their difficulties because they assume the problem is not hard, only that they are. It can even make them suspicious of care itself, because so much “help” has arrived as judgment wearing a professional tone.

This is why compassionate truth matters so much here.

People do have to change behaviors when obesity is present and health is being burdened. There is no honest way around that. Food patterns matter. Sleep matters. Movement matters. Muscle preservation matters. But if those truths are delivered without a mature understanding of how behavior actually changes, then the message becomes not only ineffective, but unfair.

Obesity is not cured by pretending habits do not matter.

It is also not well treated by pretending habits can be rebuilt by instruction alone.

The environment defeats good intentions so often because it acts at the precise points where intention is weakest. It is strongest when the person is tired. It is strongest when the person is hungry. It is strongest when the day is running late. It is strongest when the house is noisy, the budget is thin, the schedule is overloaded, and something fast feels less like indulgence than relief.

That is not the setting in which moral lectures perform well.

And the environment does not act only through food. It acts through time. Through sleep. Through commute length. Through household load. Through social norms. Through the plain fact that the body making a food decision at 8:30 p.m. is not the same body that agreed with the advice at 10:00 a.m.

A tired person is not an abstract decision-maker.

A hungry person is not an abstract decision-maker.

A parent trying to survive the evening is not an abstract decision-maker.

A shift worker on too little sleep is not an abstract decision-maker.

Any treatment plan that forgets that will keep producing avoidable disappointment.

This does not mean personal responsibility disappears. It means responsibility has to be placed inside reality. A person still has to do the work. But good medicine should be honest about what the work requires and how much friction the environment is adding to it.

That friction is not evenly distributed.

Simple advice tends to work best for people whose lives already contain buffer. Buffer time. Buffer money. Buffer sleep.

Buffer kitchen stability. Buffer social support. Buffer predictability. Buffer control over the workday. When those buffers are present, a person can sometimes make large changes from relatively modest guidance. That should be welcomed. It can be wonderful.

But those success stories should not become ammunition against the patients whose lives contain far less margin.

The more a person is constrained by fatigue, financial pressure, family load, shift work, food access, unstable schedules, or repeated exposure to convenience calories, the thinner generic advice begins to sound. Not because the advice is false. Because execution now costs more than the clinic usually admits.

That is one reason patients living with obesity so often describe feeling as though they keep failing the same test. The truth is harsher than that. They are often being handed the same underpowered treatment again and again.

So what does meaningful support look like?

It begins by becoming specific before it becomes motivational.

Meaningful support does not only say eat less. It helps restructure what, when, and how a person eats. It helps build protein into the day so fullness and muscle preservation are not left to chance. It pays attention to beverages, because liquid calories can quietly do much of the damage. It helps identify the meals that keep disappearing and the hours that keep turning into opportunistic snacking. It favors food patterns strong enough to survive hunger, not just impressive enough to sound disciplined in a clinic note.

Meaningful support also becomes realistic before it becomes idealized.

It does not assume that every patient has time for elaborate meal prep, a perfect grocery routine, or a quiet hour for the gym. It is willing to use practical foods, simple structures, partial solutions, and incremental gains. It understands that a person does not need a photographable lifestyle. A person needs a livable one.

That matters for movement too. Move more is not useless, but it is still too vague to carry much force on its own. Meaningful support turns movement into something smaller, clearer, and more repeatable. A walk after dinner. Two short strength sessions. A plan for weekends. A step goal that actually fits the body and schedule. Chair rises. Resistance bands. Stairs. Dumbbells in the corner of a room. Some way of sending the body the message that muscle still matters.

The same is true for sleep and recovery. Generic advice often treats eating as if it were independent from restoration. Meaningful support does not make that mistake. It asks whether the patient is sleeping enough to have a fair fight with appetite. It asks whether sleep apnea may be sabotaging recovery. It asks where the week is borrowing from the night. It recognizes that a person who is chronically under-recovered may need a more defensive food plan, more structure around late-day decisions, and more compassion around why the difficult hour keeps remaining difficult.

Meaningful support is also repeated.

A real obesity program cannot be only an annual warning. It has to return. It has to reassess. It has to strengthen what is working and redesign what is failing. For some patients that may come through an obesity medicine clinic. For some through a registered dietitian. For some through group visits, digital check-ins, health coaching, family support, or a good primary care relationship that treats obesity with real continuity. The method can vary.

The principle does not.

Support has to be close enough, often enough, and practical enough to compete with daily life.

That is not a small demand. It is one reason the healthcare system has often underdelivered in this space. Many clinicians are trying hard inside short visits, thin reimbursement, fragmented systems, and too little protected time for the intensity of counseling and follow-up this disease actually deserves. This is not mainly an indictment of individual clinicians. It is an indictment of a care model that has too often confused brief counseling with long-term treatment.

A field cannot call obesity chronic, relapsing, multifactorial, biologically defended, and environmentally reinforced, then act as though a few minutes of advice should usually be enough.

That is not scientific seriousness. It is therapeutic wishfulness.

The issue is not that lifestyle is unimportant.

The issue is that we have often tried to practice lifestyle medicine with the clinical seriousness of a slogan.

Patients deserve better than that. They deserve knowledge, yes. They deserve truth about food, muscle, sleep, stress, and daily structure. But they also deserve architecture. They deserve support that reaches into execution rather than stopping at explanation. They deserve plans built for their real constraints rather than for an imaginary average person with endless time and calm.

They also deserve permission to stop interpreting every failed attempt as a referendum on character.

Sometimes a patient needs to hear a different sentence than the one they have been telling themselves for years.

Not, "Why can't I do this?"

But, "What kind of support would make this more doable?"

That question moves the conversation out of shame and into design. It does not make the work easy. It makes the work more honest.

And honesty matters here because behavior change is hard enough without being mystified. It is harder when the plan is vague. Harder when the environment is saturated with easy calories. Harder when sleep is thin. Harder when every meal must compete with work, parenting, fatigue, or budget strain. Harder when the household is not aligned. Harder when the treatment goal is only to weigh less and not to preserve muscle, function, and health. Harder when follow-up is absent. Harder when each setback is treated as moral failure rather than expected friction.

Once those realities are named, advice begins to take its proper place.

Advice matters.

It is not enough.

That is the chapter's central claim, and it should not be heard as pessimism. It is actually a call to greater seriousness. A condition this common, this burdensome, and this entangled with modern life should never have been managed mainly through generalities. Patients do not need less truth. They need stronger delivery of the truth. They need treatment that helps them live the advice, not merely admire it from the exam room.

This is also where the chapter must make one more distinction.

Advice alone fails not because food and movement are irrelevant.

Advice alone fails because biology and environment are often stronger than instruction.

That sentence matters because it keeps us from making the wrong correction. If lifestyle advice is weak, the answer is not to abandon lifestyle. The answer is to stop mistaking minimal lifestyle counseling for full obesity care. Food structure still matters. Protein still matters. Strength training still matters. Sleep still matters. The environment still matters. The error was not in caring about those things. The error was in thinking a few words about them would be enough.

And for some patients, even a strong behavioral structure will still not be enough by itself.

That should not be treated as scandalous. It should be treated as medicine. There are patients whose hunger remains loud, whose biology remains resistant, whose disease burden remains substantial, and whose lives remain exposed to pressures that no amount of insight can fully neutralize. For them, the right response is not to repeat the same advice with a sharper tone.

The right response is to add leverage.

That is the transition into the next part of the story.

Because when a disease is real, when the environment is powerful, and when advice by itself has proved too weak, stronger treatment is not surrender. It is not cheating. It is not the abandonment of lifestyle. It is the recognition that patients deserve more than slogans, more than blame, and more than a pamphlet sent out to fight a chronic disease alone.

When truth is real but the delivery system is weak, medicine should not become more judgmental.

It should become more effective.

That is where medication enters the conversation.

Chapter Eleven: When Medication Helps

The injection pen is small. The hopes around it are not.

That is what waits on the other side of a chapter about why advice alone fails. If the disease is real, if the environment is strong, and if brief instruction is too weak to carry the burden, then stronger treatment belongs in the conversation.

Sometimes the first sign that medication is helping is not a lower number on the scale. It is a quieter day. The constant bargaining with food softens. The next snack does not keep interrupting thought. Fullness arrives earlier. The urge loses some of its edge. A person who has spent years being told to "just control yourself" suddenly feels a little more room between impulse and action.

That feeling deserves to be taken seriously.

It is not vanity. It is not laziness. It is not a shortcut around effort. It is biology becoming more manageable.

Modern obesity medications deserve respect. They can reduce appetite, quiet constant food preoccupation, improve metabolic health, and offer real relief to people who have struggled for years. Used well, they are not cheating, not surrender, and not the abandonment of lifestyle. They are treatment.

But medication mainly helps one part of the larger problem. It often makes it easier to eat less by making biology more manageable. It does not automatically ensure enough protein, protect muscle, improve nutrient density, or repair the environment that keeps pushing people toward disease. That is why good medication care must include protein, resistance training, body-composition-minded monitoring, realistic expectations, side-effect management, and a plan for long-term use when needed.

The larger policy danger is confusing better rescue with actual reform. A country should welcome effective obesity medication without pretending that medication alone solves an environment built around cheap calories, processed food, time scarcity, chronic stress, and poor metabolic defaults. Medication can help. It cannot be the whole answer.

The public conversation has handled these medications badly. One side treats them as miracles. Another treats them as fraud. A third treats them as moral failure in injectable form. None of those reactions helps patients. These medicines are tools. Serious ones. Imperfect ones. Sometimes transformative ones. They should not be demonized. They should also not be romanticized into a complete answer for a disease with deep upstream roots.

The newer medications matter because they changed what many patients and clinicians thought was possible. They did not invent obesity pharmacotherapy, and the field is broader than the most famous brand names. Older medications still have a real place in care, and the right choice depends on the patient in front of us, not on headlines. But the newer gut-hormone-based medications changed the scale of the conversation. They made it harder to pretend that obesity care must remain trapped between lectures and blame.

What these medicines do well is not mysterious once we say it plainly. Many of them reduce hunger, increase fullness, and change how quickly food moves through the stomach. In practical terms, eating less can become less punishing. The next meal may feel less urgent. Cravings may be easier to interrupt. Some medications also improve blood sugar and other obesity-related complications. In selected patients, the field is now moving beyond weight alone and into conditions such as cardiovascular risk and obstructive sleep apnea. That matters because it reminds the culture of something medicine should have said more clearly a long time ago: this is not cosmetic theater. This is disease treatment.

That said, the best way to understand medication is to place it inside the four-line model that has guided this book from the beginning.

Quantity in calories influences body weight.

Quality of macronutrient balance, especially protein adequacy, influences body composition.

Quality of nutrient density influences health.

Environment determines how hard or easy it is to live out the first three.

Medication often helps most directly with the first line. It can make calorie quantity easier to manage because appetite gets quieter and fullness becomes more durable. It may indirectly help the second line because a person with fewer cravings can finally structure meals around protein instead of around urgency. But medication does not guarantee the second line. A low appetite can still become a low-protein appetite. It does not guarantee the third line. A smaller food volume can still be filled with nutritionally thin convenience calories. And it certainly does not repair the fourth line. The environment remains what it was: powerful, commercial, convenient, and too often metabolically hostile.

That is why medication can succeed on the scale while treatment remains incomplete.

A quieter appetite does not automatically create a better plate.

Medication can lower intake. It cannot stock a refrigerator. It cannot redesign a workday. It cannot make healthier food more affordable. It cannot automatically preserve muscle just because pounds are dropping. In fact, when appetite falls quickly, some parts of treatment become more important, not less. If a person eats much less but protein falls with it, useful lean tissue can be lost. If energy intake falls and resistance training disappears, a body can become lighter while also becoming weaker. If the little food that remains is still dominated by highly processed, low-protein, low-nutrient options, the treatment may look better than it is.

This is why medication is not the abandonment of lifestyle. In the best cases, it is what finally makes lifestyle more livable. It gives a patient a better chance to build structure. It creates leverage. It turns down some of the biological noise so that decisions can hold more often. But if that newly opened space is not used to protect protein, preserve muscle, improve nutrient density, and make the environment more workable, then part of the opportunity is lost.

Medication makes it easier to eat less.

Protein and resistance training help the body keep what matters.

That sentence should sit near the center of modern obesity care.

When calories come down, the body still needs instruction about what tissue to keep. Protein helps provide part of that instruction by supplying building material for lean tissue and improving fullness. Resistance training provides another message: this tissue is still needed. Keep it. Resistance training does not have to mean bodybuilding. It means giving muscle a reason to stay. For one person that may mean free weights. For another, resistance bands, machines, body-weight movements, chair-stands, or supervised physical therapy. The exact form matters less than the principle. A body losing fat should be given every reasonable signal to preserve strength, function, and useful tissue.

That is especially important in the age of more effective medications because rapid improvement can tempt patients and clinicians alike to worship subtraction. The number is down. The clothes fit differently. The burden feels lighter. All of that may be good. But as earlier chapters argued, a smaller body is not automatically a healthier body if the path to getting smaller strips away too much of what should have been protected.

Good medication care therefore asks more than one question.

Not only: “How much weight came off?”

Also: “How is the person functioning?”

“How strong are they?”

“What are they eating now that appetite is lower?”

“What kind of tissue is most likely being lost?”

“What complications are improving?”

“What side effects are emerging?”

“What happens if coverage breaks?”

That last question is not a footnote. It is part of the medicine. Obesity is a chronic disease. For many patients, medication works best when it is treated as long-term chronic disease care rather than as a short burst of rescue followed by wishful thinking. That does not mean every person stays on the same medication forever. Some do well long term. Some need lower doses. Some switch agents. Some stop because of side effects, pregnancy plans, preference, cost, or other clinical realities. But the false promise is the idea that a temporary pharmacologic intervention should permanently erase a chronic, biologically defended condition without ongoing support. For many patients, that is not how this disease behaves.

It is also worth saying clearly that medication does not have to be reserved only for the final moment of desperation. A humane, evidence-based approach does not force people to fail indefinitely in order to earn help. In general, medication is considered when obesity is present, or when overweight is already accompanied by meaningful weight-related complications, and when additional biological leverage would likely improve health. The decision should be individualized. Disease burden matters. Complications matter. Previous attempts matter. Patient values matter. Route matters. Risk matters. Cost matters. Pregnancy plans matter. Other medications matter. No one drug is right for everyone. No one patient profile should be flattened into a trend story.

This is also where dignity matters. No patient should be pushed toward medication because the culture is obsessed with appearance. And no patient who wants legitimate treatment should be shamed because the culture mistakes obesity care for vanity. The clinic has to be calmer and more serious than that. The goals should be health, function, burden reduction, and quality of life. Not humiliation. Not aesthetic conformity. Not panic.

Because this chapter needs to do more than argue, it should also make visible what careful medication care looks like in practice.

Practical Medication-Care Checklist

Moment	What careful care includes	Why it matters
Before the first dose	Define goals beyond the scale; review obesity-related complications, prior treatment history, current medications, pregnancy plans, major gastrointestinal symptoms, diabetes therapies, mood history, and affordability; record baseline weight, waist, blood pressure, and labs as indicated; ask about current protein intake, strength work, and day-to-day function	Medication choice should fit the patient, not the trend. A baseline makes later progress easier to judge honestly
During dose escalation	Increase slowly as tolerated; prioritize hydration; reduce meal size before skipping eating entirely; make protein visible at regular meals; keep some form of resistance training in the week; prepare for bowel changes early	Most side effects appear early, and this is also when unintentional under-eating and muscle loss can begin
Once a maintenance dose is reached	Reassess hunger, cravings, weight, waist, energy, strength, and body composition if available; review blood sugar if other diabetes medications are being used; decide whether the current dose is enough, too much, or not workable	The right dose is the one that helps health and can actually be lived with, not automatically the highest dose

Moment	What careful care includes	Why it matters
If progress stalls	Check access interruptions, protein intake, resistance training, sleep, stress, meal structure, and food environment before assuming the biology alone is the problem	A plateau does not always mean failure. Sometimes the plan needs redesign, not blame
If treatment is not helping enough	Revisit diagnosis, expectations, adherence, tolerability, complications, and alternative medication options; consider whether the patient now needs a more powerful or more durable intervention	Good care escalates thoughtfully. It does not keep repeating the same plan after it has stopped serving the patient

One of the common mistakes in practice is assuming that less appetite automatically means better nutrition. In fact, the opposite risk often appears. When appetite shrinks, food quality matters more, not less. There is less room for nutritional carelessness. A person who used to eat large amounts may now be eating much smaller volumes. That makes protein adequacy, fiber, hydration, and nutrient density more important because there is less room to accidentally get them right.

In practical terms, that often means building meals around recognizable protein-rich foods and then filling in the rest with produce, fiber-rich foods, and other healthier staples that fit the person's culture, budget, and household reality. It does not require perfection. It does require intention. If the medication is doing the work of reducing appetite, the rest of the plan has to do the work of improving what that smaller appetite is spent on.

This is also where side effects have to be handled like real medicine, not like personal weakness. Most patients who struggle early are not failing the drug. They are running into predictable physiology during initiation or dose escalation. Good clinical care anticipates that rather than acting surprised by it.

Common Side Effects and What Usually Helps

Common issue	What people often notice	What usually helps	When to call sooner
Nausea or early fullness	Feeling "too full," queasy, especially after larger meals or dose increases	Smaller meals, slower eating, less greasy or very heavy food, hydration, and sometimes a slower titration pace	If the symptom is severe, persistent, or making eating and drinking difficult
Vomiting or poor intake	Trouble keeping food down, fear of eating, fast fatigue	Fluids, temporary simplification of meals, dose reassessment with the prescribing clinician	If fluids cannot be kept down, signs of dehydration appear, or weakness escalates
Constipation	Hard stools, less frequent stools, bloating, abdominal discomfort	Early attention to fluids, walking, fiber as tolerated, and bowel support if appropriate	If abdominal pain is increasing, constipation is severe, or the person is not passing stool or gas normally
Diarrhea	Loose stools, urgency, cramping	Hydration, simpler meals, review of high-fat triggers, and dose/tolerance reassessment	If diarrhea is persistent, severe, or causing dehydration
Reflux, burping, bloating	Heartburn, pressure, uncomfortable fullness, belching	Smaller portions, slower eating, not lying down right after meals, review of trigger foods	If pain is severe, symptoms are progressive, or eating becomes very difficult
Red-flag symptoms	Severe persistent abdominal pain, marked dehydration, faintness, jaundice, inability to eat or drink, worsening mood symptoms, or unusual clinical change	These are not "push through it" symptoms	Contact the treating clinician promptly or seek urgent care or emergency department care depending on severity

Good side-effect management also means remembering that forcing a patient upward through dose escalation is not the same thing as practicing strong medicine. Sometimes the wiser move is slower titration. Sometimes it is holding at a lower dose that still provides meaningful benefit. Sometimes it is changing medications entirely. The goal is not to prove toughness. The goal is to improve health.

Monitoring should reflect that same seriousness.

A Practical Monitoring Rhythm

Timing	Main questions	What to look for
Baseline	Is medication appropriate, and what kind of success are we actually aiming for?	Weight, waist, blood pressure, relevant labs, complications, current eating pattern, protein intake, strength/function, medications, pregnancy plans, access barriers
Early follow-up	Is the patient tolerating initiation, and is the plan still nutritionally sound?	Nausea, bowel changes, hydration, ability to meet protein goals, blood sugar if relevant, adherence, affordability, technique, emotional response to treatment
After reaching a therapeutic dose	Is the medication truly helping, and what kind of weight is likely being lost?	Weight trend, waist trend, hunger/craving changes, energy, strength, functional markers, body composition if available, complications improving or not
Ongoing maintenance	Is this still the right medication, at the right dose, for the right goal?	Plateaus, regain, access interruptions, side effects, sustained protein and activity patterns, quality of life, need for dose change, switch, or escalation
Before surgery, pregnancy, or major plan changes	Does the medication plan need to be modified or paused?	Pregnancy plans, perioperative instructions, dehydration risk, oral medication considerations, and the need for close coordination with the full care team

The body-composition point deserves one more emphasis because it is one of the most neglected parts of this entire national conversation. If a sophisticated body composition tool is available, it can be useful. If it is not, that does not excuse the clinic from asking better questions. Waist size, strength, physical function, energy, signs of undernourishment, dietary protein, and the patient's lived capacity all give clues about whether treatment is improving health or just dropping mass. The perfect measurement is not required. Attention is required.

A patient who has lost weight but feels markedly weaker, is eating very little protein, has abandoned resistance work, and cannot climb stairs as well as before should not be congratulated too quickly. A patient whose weight loss is slower than expected but whose waist is improving, blood sugar is better, sleep is better, joint burden is lighter, appetite is calmer, and strength is holding may be doing very well indeed.

The scale records change.

Medicine has to decide what kind of change it was.

Medication Decision Pathway

Pathway point	Action or decision	Next move
1. Comprehensive assessment	Review disease burden, complications, goals, prior treatment, access, current medication list, pregnancy considerations when relevant, and the patient's nutrition, movement, sleep, stress, and functional baseline.	Ask: **Is medication appropriate?**
2A. If no, or not now	Strengthen non-drug care: nutrition structure, protein, movement, sleep, stress, and environmental supports.	Reassess over time and revisit medication if disease burden, goals, or circumstances change.
2B. If yes	Choose medication through shared decision-making: expected benefit, risk, route, cost, coverage, preference, and clinical fit.	Build the care plan before the first dose.
3. Build the care plan first	Include protein, hydration, resistance training, body-composition-minded monitoring, and a side-effect plan.	Start low and titrate as tolerated.
4. Early follow-up	Ask: **Is the patient tolerating the medication?**	If yes, continue and reassess. If no, slow titration, use a lower dose, manage side effects, or reconsider the medication.

Pathway point	Action or decision	Next move
5A. If still not workable	Stop or switch medication and rebuild the plan around the patient's goals, risks, and preferences.	Return to shared decision-making rather than forcing a failing plan.
5B. If workable	Continue and reassess.	Monitor weight, waist, strength, function, protein intake, and body composition if available.
6. Health benefit review	Ask: **Is there meaningful health benefit?**	If yes, continue long-term care, expect plateaus, and adjust over time.
7. If no, or not enough	Check adherence, access, food quality, protein, resistance training, sleep, and stress before assuming the medication alone is the problem.	Ask: **Does the patient need more leverage or a more durable option?**
8A. If no	Continue long-term care and refine the plan.	Keep monitoring and strengthening the supports that are working.
8B. If yes	Discuss next-level treatment, including metabolic surgery when appropriate.	Bridge into a respectful, medically serious conversation about surgical options.

Expectation-setting matters because unrealistic hope can injure treatment just as much as cynicism can. Not every patient gets a dramatic result. Response varies. Some people feel an early shift in appetite. Others need time. Some have meaningful benefit at lower doses. Others do not tolerate escalation well. Some improve in ways the scale only partially captures. Others plateau sooner than they expected. None of this means nothing is happening. But it does mean that medication should be framed honestly from the beginning.

A good opening conversation usually includes several truths at once.

The medication may help substantially.

It may also cause side effects.

The dose may need patience.

The best endpoint is not only a smaller body, but a healthier one.

The plan will work better if protein, strength, and food quality are protected.

Stopping later may lead to regain.

Long-term use may be reasonable for a chronic disease.

And no patient should interpret the need for ongoing treatment as a moral defeat.

That last part matters because the culture remains confused about what counts as legitimate help. We do not usually tell patients with high blood pressure that needing a medication proves they have failed characterologically. We do not tell patients with asthma that using a controller medication is cheating because breathing should be possible without assistance. Obesity deserves the same medical seriousness. Using an evidence-based medication for a chronic disease is not a confession of weakness. It is a treatment decision.

But neither should medication be turned into a new way of minimizing the larger truth. The leadership mistake would be to let downstream success become upstream excuse. A country should not congratulate itself for becoming better at suppressing appetite while remaining careless about the food system, the cheap-calorie economy, the time pressures, and the daily design that keep feeding the disease.

Downstream treatment deserves respect.

Downstream treatment is not upstream repair.

That distinction becomes even more important once access enters the picture. The access problem is not a side issue in obesity medicine. It is one of its central ethical questions. These medications can be expensive. Coverage rules have often been inconsistent. Prior authorization requirements can be exhausting. Step therapy, plan exclusions, and administrative churn can break continuity. For some patients, the start of treatment is easier than the staying on it. That is not a minor inconvenience. For a chronic disease, interruption is a clinical event.

Coverage interruptions are not just paperwork.

They are biology.

If a treatment works best when sustained, then repeated denial, delay, or discontinuity can set patients up for unnecessary regain, frustration, and shame. The people most able to privately absorb cost and navigate bureaucratic friction should not be the only ones able to access modern obesity care. A system that offers real leverage only to the affluent is not practicing equitable medicine.

The same pressure has pushed some patients toward loosely marketed, unapproved, or casually sourced alternatives. That is not a trivial development. Safety, quality control, dosing accuracy, and proper clinical supervision matter. A medication should begin inside a real clinical relationship, not inside a loophole, a social-media feed, or a payment page that is pretending supervision is the same thing as care.

And even if access were perfect tomorrow, another ethical problem would remain. If we are willing to fund powerful downstream treatment, we should not act as though the nutrition support that makes treatment safer and more effective is optional or decorative. The same goes for strength-preserving physical activity support, body-composition-minded follow-up, and the food quality required when appetite has become smaller. A healthcare system that will pay for an expensive rescue but not help patients build a metabolically better daily pattern is still thinking too narrowly.

That argument will return later in this book in a more upstream form. For now, it is enough to say this: medication works best when it is supported by real care, and real care should not end at the prescription.

This is why the national future cannot be medication versus reform. It has to be medication and reform, held in the right order. We should want excellent treatment for the patient in front of us. We should also refuse to mistake excellent treatment for a solved upstream problem. Those are not competing moral duties. They are the same duty seen at two distances.

Close up, the physician helps the person who is suffering now.

At a wider angle, the physician should also help ask why so many people needed rescue in the first place.

That is the real governing tension of this chapter. Medication can be one of the best tools modern obesity medicine has gained. It can reduce suffering. It can improve health. It can create relief where years of instructions did not. It belongs in serious care. But if the country keeps manufacturing obesity efficiently and then congratulates itself for getting better at pharmacologic rescue, it will still be practicing an incomplete form of honesty.

Medication can help.

It can help a great deal.

It is still downstream.

And even with excellent medical care, some patients need more leverage than medication can provide, cannot tolerate the drugs well enough, or need a more durable intervention than medication alone can reliably deliver. That should not be read as scandal, and it should not be read as failure. It should be read as medicine.

That is where the next chapter begins.

Because when medication helps, it deserves respect.

And when surgery helps, it deserves the same.

Chapter Twelve: When Surgery Helps

It is still dark outside. In a preoperative bay, a person sits in a hospital gown with an IV in the arm and a plastic bag holding the clothes they wore in from the parking garage. The stomach has been empty since midnight. The mind has not. Hope is in the room, but so are fear, blood pressure cuffs, paperwork, and the quiet understanding that something serious is about to happen.

No one looking closely at that moment should call it the easy way out.

And yet that is one of the phrases people living with obesity still hear when surgery enters the conversation. The phrase tells us almost nothing about surgery. It tells us a great deal about the way obesity has been moralized in public life.

The last chapter argued that medication deserves respect. Surgery does too. That should not be controversial. In the culture we actually live in, it still is.

This chapter has to hold two truths together. Bariatric and metabolic surgery can be transformative for selected patients. It can reduce disease burden, improve quality of life, and change the trajectory of a life that has been getting steadily smaller under the burden of obesity and its complications. It deserves respect, not dismissal.

The second truth is just as important. Surgery is a rescue tool, not the center of a national prevention strategy. A society should not need rescue at the scale its own design is creating. A country cannot operate its way out of a food environment that keeps manufacturing disease.

What most people casually call weight-loss surgery is more accurately described as bariatric or metabolic surgery. The ordinary label is understandable, but it is incomplete. These operations certainly can produce substantial weight loss. But the word weight is still too narrow for what is actually happening.

The word metabolic matters.

These procedures do more than make the stomach smaller. They change the physiology surrounding hunger, fullness, eating behavior, and blood sugar regulation. People often imagine surgery as a purely mechanical intervention, as if the whole effect were simply that a patient can no longer eat as much. That is part of the story. It is not the whole story.

A sleeve gastrectomy removes a large portion of the stomach. A gastric bypass creates a much smaller stomach pouch and reroutes part of the digestive tract. Different operations work through somewhat different balances of restriction, absorption, and hormonal change. A reader does not need to memorize the anatomy to understand the larger point. These operations alter the conversation between the gut, the brain, and the rest of metabolism.

Meals become smaller. Fullness often arrives sooner. Hunger often softens. Food can feel different in the body. Blood sugar regulation may improve, sometimes before dramatic visible weight loss has even had time to occur. That is one reason the term metabolic surgery is not a marketing phrase. It reflects the fact that these operations are acting on disease biology, not just on body size.

For the right patient, that biologic shift can be profound.

Type 2 diabetes may improve dramatically. Sleep apnea may improve. Blood pressure burden may lessen. Fatty liver disease may improve. Joint strain often becomes lighter as excess body fat comes down. Mobility can improve. Stamina can improve. The body can become easier to live in again.

Sometimes the most meaningful result is not a number on the scale at all. It is being able to tie shoes without struggling for breath. It is rising from the floor with less effort. It is walking through an airport with less pain. It is sleeping more safely. It is keeping up with children or grandchildren. It is no longer organizing every day around physical and metabolic burdens that have become harder and harder to carry.

That matters because this book has already argued that weight is not the same as health. Surgery does not disprove that. It reinforces it. The best outcome after surgery is not merely that the body is smaller. The best outcome is that disease burden is lower, function is better, and life has widened.

This is also why surgery should never be discussed as a cosmetic shortcut. It is not a beauty procedure for people who have become impatient with the mirror. It is a serious treatment for a serious disease.

That said, surgery is powerful. It is not magic.

Chronic disease does not disappear as a category simply because anatomy has changed. Some patients later need medication. Some experience plateaus. Some regain some weight. Some continue to live under strong environmental pressure from the same cheap calories, same stress, same long workdays, and same food landscape that helped create the disease in the first place. None of that means surgery was illegitimate. It means obesity remained what it has been all along: a chronic disease living inside a chronic environment.

In that sense, surgery changes leverage. It changes how much help the biology is giving the patient. It does not turn the patient into someone who no longer needs care, structure, or follow-up.

A serious chapter on surgery therefore has to resist two opposite mistakes. The first is treating surgery as a defeat reserved for people who somehow lacked discipline. The second is treating it as a casual solution for anyone unhappy with the scale. Good care does neither.

The right question is not who deserves surgery.

The right question is who is likely to benefit from it safely, meaningfully, and sustainably.

In general, surgery becomes more important as obesity becomes more severe, metabolic and mechanical complications accumulate, function worsens, and lesser tools have not been enough. A person with substantial excess adiposity, worsening diabetes, sleep apnea, increasing liver fat, progressive joint pain, major mobility limits, or a rising physical burden may be living with a level of disease that deserves stronger therapy.

This is not about making people earn surgery by suffering a little longer.

Patients do not need to prove moral seriousness by staying sicker than necessary.

That point matters because obesity care has too often required patients to perform years of struggle before more effective treatment is considered legitimate. They try repeated dietary approaches. They try exercise plans that cannot outpace the biology and the environment. They blame themselves. They lose and regain. Blood sugar rises. Sleep worsens. Pain grows. Then, only after long frustration, surgery is finally spoken of as though it were the last acceptable step after the culture has been reassured that the patient tried hard enough.

That is not a medically mature way to think.

Surgery should be considered when the disease burden and the likely benefit justify it, not only when the patient has accumulated enough shame to make the public feel comfortable. A person does not become more worthy of help by waiting longer.

At the same time, thoughtful evaluation matters. Not because patients need to be judged. Because real surgery deserves real preparation.

A good program looks at the whole person and the whole disease. Severity matters, of course. But so do diabetes burden, sleep-disordered breathing, reflux, liver disease, nutritional risk, prior abdominal operations, medications, pregnancy plans, physical function, emotional readiness, and the patient's own goals and preferences. A person with significant reflux, for example, may not face the same surgical decision as a person without it. A patient with advanced diabetes may not face exactly the same decision as someone whose main burden is mechanical and functional. The operation should fit the patient. The patient should not be forced to fit an ideology.

This is also one reason there is no prize for turning medication and surgery into opposing camps. Some patients will choose medication instead of surgery. Some will use medication as a bridge to surgery. Some will later benefit from medication after surgery. These are not rival religions. They are tools. The mature question in obesity medicine is not Which tribe are you in? It is What level of treatment does this disease now require?

Respect for surgery also means refusing to romanticize it.

Every real operation carries real risk. Bleeding, infection, blood clots, leaks, dehydration, and longer-term nutritional problems are not imaginary. No honest physician should turn surgery into something casual merely to defend it from stigma. Respect is not the same thing as cheerleading. Respect tells the truth about benefits and burdens at the same time.

The operation takes hours. The adaptation takes much longer.

Meals become smaller. Eating too fast usually becomes self-punishing. Protein has to become intentional. Fluids matter. Vitamins and minerals may need lifelong supplementation and monitoring, especially depending on the procedure. Laboratory follow-up matters. Ongoing medical follow-up matters. The scars may be small. The commitment is not.

That commitment is one more reason the phrase easy way out is so unserious. Surgery asks a great deal of the patient. It asks preoperative appointments, education, anesthesia, recovery, altered eating, long-term follow-up, and a willingness to care for the body differently afterward. Calling that easy after years of disease burden is not insight. It is disrespect.

The earlier chapters of this book still apply after surgery. A smaller stomach does not remove the importance of protein. Rapid weight loss can still cost muscle if protein intake falls too low and resistance training disappears. The scale may celebrate while the body quietly weakens.

That is why serious postoperative care keeps returning to the same target this book has insisted on from the beginning: lose fat, keep muscle, preserve function.

After surgery, each bite often has to work harder. There is less room for nutritional carelessness. If appetite is lower and meal volume is smaller, then protein adequacy and nutrient density become even more important. A patient can lose a striking amount of weight and still do so in a way that underprotects lean mass if the food structure is poor. A good surgical program does more than schedule an operation. It teaches, monitors, and keeps caring long after the incisions heal.

This is also where the four-line model stays useful.

Surgery can powerfully influence calorie quantity. It can create new room to improve body composition if protein and resistance training are taken seriously. It can improve nutrient density if smaller meals become more intentional. But it does not repair the fourth line. It does not rewrite the environment.

The patient still goes home to the same prices, the same convenience culture, the same work schedule, the same family stress, the same school food, the same late-night food delivery apps, the same sleep pressures, and the same national defaults. Surgery changes the body. The environment is waiting unchanged.

That truth matters for another reason too. Some of the social and emotional work begins after the operation, not before it.

The body changes. Appetite changes. Portions change. Family routines around food may need to change. Expectations can become unrealistic. Other people may respond with curiosity, admiration, discomfort, or judgment. A person may feel relief and vulnerability at the same time. Good care leaves room for that complexity. Surgery is not only an anatomical event. It is a life event.

All of this makes the stigma around surgery look even thinner than it already did.

The cultural contempt directed at bariatric surgery is misguided for two opposite reasons. It understates what the patient has already carried, and it understates what the surgery itself actually asks.

Many people who pursue surgery have already spent years trying to solve the disease with advice, restriction, gym memberships, private guilt, repeated self-surveillance, and the exhausting cycle of hope followed by regain. They arrive not because effort was absent. They arrive because effort alone was not enough against severe disease biology and a strong environment.

Some have watched diabetes worsen while they tried to be more disciplined. Some have watched sleep become noisier and less safe. Some have felt their knees, hips, or back carry more burden than they can comfortably tolerate. Some have lived for years under the humiliation of pretending the struggle must reflect a flaw of character. By the time surgery is considered, many patients have already given the culture more proof of effort than the culture had any right to demand.

Then the same culture wants to call surgery cheating.

There is something deeply revealing in that response.

We do not usually tell a patient with severe coronary disease that accepting a stent is weakness. We do not tell a person who needs a hip replacement that the honorable path is to limp for five more years. We do not tell a patient with cataracts that surgery is morally inferior to seeing poorly for longer. Yet obesity remains one of the few conditions in which people are still asked to defend themselves for using effective treatment.

There is nothing morally elevated about untreated disease.

Patients do not owe the public a performance of suffering before they are allowed relief.

This is where medicine has to be better than the culture around it. A physician may discuss risk. A physician may recommend for or against surgery in a specific case. A physician may say that one patient needs medication, another needs surgery, and a third needs continued structured non-surgical care. All of that can be appropriate. What should not happen is moral suspicion disguised as clinical judgment.

If healthcare professionals speak about metabolic surgery as failure, desperation, or personal weakness rather than as a legitimate therapy, we teach patients to delay care they may genuinely need. We push them back toward shame. We make the disease heavier before we ever make it lighter.

A humane field should reject that.

It should also reject the strange idea that "natural" is always the morally superior path. Obesity is not noble because it is untreated. A person is not more virtuous because they continue to lose the same fight against severe disease with weaker tools. Medicine exists because nature is often not enough. There is nothing unserious about using treatment when treatment is indicated.

Still, a chapter like this would become incomplete if respect for surgery turned into national complacency.

Because surgery can be so effective for selected patients, the country may be tempted to treat it as proof that the obesity problem is being handled well enough. It is not.

Rescue is not redesign.

By the time a patient reaches an operating room, years of the upstream story have already acted. The engineered-food environment has acted. The cheap-calorie economy has acted. Short sleep has acted. Chronic stress has acted. Childhood exposure has acted. Advice without enough structure has acted. The operation enters the story after the river has been flowing for a long time.

A procedure can change anatomy in a morning. It cannot change grocery prices waiting when the patient gets home. It cannot remove low-nutrient, highly processed foods from school hallways. It cannot shorten commutes, protect sleep, or redesign the break room. It cannot by itself make vegetables, fruit, and quality protein easier to buy than the cheap calories that helped produce the disease in the first place.

That is why a nation cannot build enough operating rooms to solve what grocery aisles, school food, short sleep, chronic stress, and cheap calories keep producing.

This is not an argument against surgery. It is an argument against letting surgery become an alibi.

Even in a healthier society, some patients would still need surgical help. Biology would still vary. Severe obesity would still exist. Genetics would still matter. Some patients would still need a level of metabolic leverage that food counseling, medication, and good intentions could not fully provide. The argument is not that surgery should disappear. The argument is that a decent society should stop acting as though rescue alone counts as strategy.

In fact, the stronger our rescue tools become, the harder the upstream question should be to avoid.

If surgery can dramatically reduce disease burden for the right patient, then we should be grateful such a tool exists. We should also ask, with greater urgency rather than less, why so many people are getting pushed so far downstream before meaningful leverage appears. The better question is not whether surgery is too aggressive. The better question is why upstream prevention has been so timid.

That question belongs not only to policymakers, but to physicians. If we are serious about obesity medicine as a field, we cannot limit ourselves to documenting who needs rescue after the fact. We have to become more willing to challenge the conditions that keep producing the next wave of patients.

This matters economically as well as morally. A system that can justify paying for hospital care, anesthesia, surgeons, operating rooms, follow-up, and the management of downstream complications should at least be willing to think seriously about the conditions it is financing around. It is a strange arrangement when the system is more comfortable paying for late-stage rescue than helping patients gain reliable access to the food that would make rescue less necessary and postoperative success easier to sustain.

That mismatch becomes even starker after surgery. Once a patient has undergone a life-changing operation, the very things that matter most afterward are often the things our system still treats as optional or private. Protein quality matters. Nutrient density matters. Healthier staples matter. Follow-up matters. The patient's food environment still matters. A body that can no longer live on large volumes still needs access to foods that are metabolically worth eating.

A system willing to pay for rescue should not behave as though postoperative nutrition is merely a matter of private virtue. Nor should it behave as though healthier food access before surgery is some lifestyle luxury floating outside real medical care. Food is not an accessory to metabolic health. It is one of its daily conditions.

This is where the chapter's two truths come back together.

Surgery can be life-changing. For the right patient, it can reduce suffering in ways that no lecture ever could. It can interrupt a disease trajectory that has been worsening for years. It belongs inside serious obesity medicine. It should be respected, supported, and discussed without mockery.

But surgery should never become the center of the national narrative. If the country treats bariatric surgery as the main answer while leaving the disease-producing environment largely intact, then the country is not solving obesity. It is managing the consequences of an upstream failure with increasing downstream skill.

That is better than neglect. It is still not enough.

A society that offers excellent surgery to people who need it is doing something good. A society that offers surgery while leaving cheap disease-promoting calories easier to buy than vegetables, fruit, and quality protein is still not thinking upstream enough.

Surgery is powerful for the right patient. It can be transformative. It can widen life again. It should never be mocked, and it should never be minimized.

But it should also never become an excuse for leaving the deeper problem untouched.

Surgery is powerful rescue. It should never excuse upstream failure. If the healthcare system can justify paying for operating rooms after disease is established, it should be willing to think much more seriously about helping patients access vegetables, fruit, quality protein, and healthier staple foods before and after that point.

The prescription pad must go upstream.

Chapter Thirteen: The Prescription Pad Must Go Upstream

A patient sits in front of me, holding a new prescription for an expensive injectable medication.

Insurance will likely cover it. Prior authorization will be submitted. The system will mobilize. The pharmacy will process it. The medication will be refrigerated, dispensed, and administered with clinical precision.

It may cost thousands of dollars a year.

And yet that same patient may struggle to afford a consistent supply of vegetables, fruit, quality protein, and healthier staple foods.

We have built a healthcare system that can finance rescue at scale.

We have not yet built one that consistently finances prevention.

That imbalance is no longer defensible.

Earlier in this book, we made room for medications. We made room for surgery. We told the truth about why advice alone fails. We acknowledged the power of modern pharmacotherapy and the real transformation it can bring to patients who have struggled for years.

Now we have to say something equally clear.

If a prescription can unlock coverage for an expensive injectable, a prescription should also be able to unlock access to vegetables, fruit, quality protein, and a diet that does not predictably worsen disease.

That sentence is not symbolic.

It is economic.

It is clinical.

It is moral.

And it is long overdue.

Obesity medicine has spent decades working downstream. We have documented rising blood sugar, fatty liver, sleep apnea, hypertension, joint strain, and metabolic disease. We have treated the consequences with skill and growing sophistication. We have added medications. We have refined surgery. We have improved follow-up.

But while we have been refining rescue, the food environment has continued producing new disease upstream.

This chapter is about moving the prescription pad into that upstream space.

Food belongs in medical treatment.

That statement should not be controversial. Every physician understands, at least in theory, that nutrition shapes blood sugar, blood pressure, lipid levels, liver health, inflammation, body composition, and long-term disease risk. We counsel patients about food every day. We write handouts. We refer to dietitians. We warn about sugary drinks and ultra-processed diets.

But counseling without economic leverage is often too weak against structural exposure.

A patient may fully understand that adequate protein supports muscle preservation. They may understand that minimally processed foods support nutrient density. They may understand that ultra-processed, hyper-palatable convenience food makes overconsumption easier.

Understanding does not automatically produce access.

Access costs money. Access costs time. Access competes with shelf life, transport, neighborhood retail patterns, budget constraints, and the cheap-calorie economy we examined earlier in this book.

And here is the uncomfortable truth.

The healthcare system routinely spends extraordinary sums managing diseases that are strongly influenced by diet. It pays for insulin. It pays for antihypertensives. It pays for cholesterol-lowering agents. It pays for advanced imaging. It pays for dialysis. It pays for bariatric surgery. It pays for high-cost obesity medications. It pays for hospitalizations. It pays for procedures.

It hesitates, however, to pay directly for food.

We treat food as lifestyle. We treat medication as medicine.

Biology does not recognize that distinction.

The pancreas does not know whether glucose rose because the system financed ultra-processed food exposure for decades but refused to subsidize nutrient-dense alternatives. The liver does not care whether fatty infiltration occurred in a world where cheap calories were easier to afford than quality protein and fresh produce. The knee does not care whether excess weight accumulated in an environment saturated with hyper-palatable convenience food.

The body responds to exposure, regardless of how the system categorizes it.

If we accept that modern obesity is partly a predictable result of a cheap-calorie economy, then helping patients access better food is not charity.

It is rational medical intervention.

Some will say that physicians should not be in the business of prescribing groceries. That food is a personal matter. That markets should determine supply and demand. That insurance exists to pay for medical services, not shopping lists.

But this objection misunderstands what is being proposed.

No one is asking physicians to micromanage dinner. We are asking that medically indicated, evidence-based nutritional support be treated as a legitimate health intervention when disease risk is present.

We already accept this logic in other contexts.

We cover cardiac rehabilitation after a heart attack. We cover insulin for diabetes. We cover inhalers for asthma. We cover medications for hypertension. We cover dialysis for kidney failure. We cover surgery when joints fail.

Why is it unreasonable to cover medically tailored nutrition when excess adiposity, insulin resistance, increased liver fat, or metabolic syndrome are already present?

The economic case is straightforward.

Downstream treatment is expensive.

Upstream food intervention, done intelligently, may cost far less.

The moral case is equally clear.

If we are willing to pay for treatment after disease has developed, we should at least consider paying for interventions that reduce the probability or severity of that disease in the first place.

This is not theoretical. Around the country, small but growing programs are testing variations of what this could look like: produce prescriptions, medically tailored meal programs, food pharmacies embedded in clinics, healthy-food benefit cards, partnerships between healthcare systems and local grocers, nutrition-support programs for patients with diabetes, heart failure, kidney disease, and obesity.

The early lessons are not that food cures everything.

They are that access changes behavior when paired with structure.

When a patient receives not just advice but actual support to obtain vegetables, fruit, protein-rich foods, and healthier staples, adherence becomes less abstract. The friction decreases. The grocery aisle becomes less adversarial. The budget stretches differently. The refrigerator looks different. The late-week panic looks different.

This is the fourth line of the model applied directly.

Environment determines how hard or easy it is to live out the first three.

If the environment includes structured, subsidized access to healthier food, adherence becomes more plausible.

If the environment includes only cheap, ultra-processed calories and lectures about willpower, adherence becomes heroism.

Heroism is not a scalable public-health strategy.

Some critics worry that prescribing food creates dependency or undermines personal responsibility. But this argument collapses under scrutiny.

We do not accuse patients of dependency when we prescribe statins. We do not accuse them of moral weakness when we authorize sleep apnea equipment. We do not accuse them of irresponsibility when we cover bariatric surgery. We recognize that disease requires support.

Healthy-food access is not indulgence.

It is infrastructure.

And if we are honest, the system already subsidizes food—just not in a way aligned with metabolic health. Agricultural policy, commodity pricing, supply chains, marketing incentives, and retail structures all shape what is cheap and what is expensive. The current arrangement often makes calorie-dense, shelf-stable, ultra-processed products cheaper and more durable than fresher, protein-rich, fiber-rich alternatives.

That is not an accident of nature. It is a product of economic design.

Markets are engines. Incentives determine what those engines produce.

If the strongest incentives reward shelf life, margin, and cheap calories, the engine will produce more of them.

If incentives begin rewarding nutrient density, protein adequacy, and healthier defaults at scale, the engine can move in a different direction.

Physicians should not stand outside that conversation.

Obesity medicine has a responsibility not only to treat the patient in front of us, but to question the conditions that keep producing the next patient.

That responsibility does not require hostility toward business. It requires literacy about incentives.

Consider the asymmetry we have normalized.

A patient with obesity and insulin resistance can receive a prescription for an injectable medication that may cost thousands of dollars annually. Insurance may approve it. The healthcare system may absorb a substantial share of the cost.

That same patient may not be able to afford consistent access to high-quality protein, fresh produce, and minimally processed staples without meaningful strain.

We have built coverage pathways for pharmacology.

We have not built equally serious coverage pathways for food.

That is an imbalance of priorities, not a law of physics.

The prescription pad is a powerful economic instrument. It can unlock coverage, trigger reimbursement, and reshape access. For too long, we have confined its use to pills and procedures.

It is time to expand its reach.

This does not mean writing a vague note that says "eat better." It means developing structured programs where physicians can prescribe medically indicated nutrition support that is redeemable, accountable, and outcome-oriented.

Imagine a patient with obesity and prediabetes receiving a structured produce and protein benefit linked to clinical follow-up.

Imagine a patient on an appetite-lowering medication being supported with food access that emphasizes protein adequacy and nutrient density, protecting muscle and improving body composition rather than simply shrinking the scale.

Imagine a patient with fatty liver disease being enrolled in a medically tailored nutrition program as a core part of treatment rather than as an optional add-on.

Imagine insurers recognizing that covering a portion of healthier food costs for high-risk patients is a rational investment compared with years of downstream pharmacotherapy and complication management.

This is not fantasy.

It is alignment.

Alignment between what we know biologically and what we finance economically.

Some will argue that physicians should stay in their lane, that food policy is political, that economics is someone else's domain.

But obesity is already political. Food pricing is already political. Insurance coverage is already political. Agricultural subsidy is already political. Marketing to children is already political.

The only question is whether physicians will participate intelligently in shaping those forces or remain confined to documenting their consequences.

Obesity medicine cannot remain content to operate only at the bottom of the cliff.

We have to be willing to ask why so many people are falling.

Healthy-food prescriptions are not about policing taste. They are about reducing predictable harm. They are about acknowledging that the cheap-calorie economy we described earlier is not a neutral background. It is a metabolic driver.

And drivers can be countered.

The economics of food access also intersect with dignity. Telling a patient to eat more vegetables while knowing those vegetables are financially and logistically harder to obtain than processed alternatives creates quiet moral tension. The advice is correct. The execution is expensive.

When physicians can pair nutritional guidance with tangible access support, the conversation shifts. It becomes less accusatory and more collaborative. It says, in effect, we are not only asking you to change; we are helping change the conditions around you.

That is what serious chronic-disease management looks like.

It is also worth stating plainly that food intervention should not be reserved only for the lowest-income patients. Middle-income households also experience time poverty, budget pressure, and food-environment saturation. The problem is not only income; it is exposure. Programs may need to be targeted, scaled, and economically designed carefully, but the principle is broad: when diet is a major driver of disease, diet should be part of covered treatment.

This does not absolve individuals of responsibility. It strengthens their capacity to act.

Personal agency matters. It always will. But agency without access is fragile. Agency supported by structure is durable.

If we can spend thousands per year on medications that manage appetite, we should be willing to spend a fraction of that on food access that supports protein adequacy, nutrient density, and metabolic stability.

If we can finance dialysis after kidney failure, we should consider financing nutrition support that reduces progression of metabolic disease.

If we can reimburse for bariatric surgery when indicated, we should be willing to reimburse for upstream nutritional intervention before the disease becomes severe.

Upstream obesity medicine should help patients afford healthier food, not only afford treatment after unhealthy food has already done the damage.

That is the chapter's central claim.

And it is not anti-medication.

It is pro-balance.

Medications and surgery deserve their place. They save lives. They restore function. They relieve suffering. But they are downstream tools.

Food is daily exposure.

If daily exposure remains structurally misaligned with metabolic health, we will keep treating the consequences at scale.

The prescription pad can do more than manage blood pressure and blood sugar.

It can help shape the economic realities that patients live inside.

It can send a signal to insurers that food is not peripheral.

It can send a signal to policymakers that healthcare dollars should not ignore upstream leverage.

It can send a signal to the market that nutrient density and metabolic protection are worthy of structural support.

The deeper question is not feasibility alone.

It is whether we are willing to test, measure, and scale what works.

Physicians hold more influence than we sometimes admit. We write guidelines. We sit on advisory panels. We advise insurers. We shape benefit design. We speak to employers. We testify before policymakers. We help define what counts as medically necessary.

If obesity is a disease shaped heavily by food environment, then medically meaningful food access is not a luxury.

It is part of care.

The country does not need less treatment. It needs wider treatment.

Treatment that still honors medication and surgery when appropriate.

Treatment that still respects patient agency.

Treatment that still tells the truth about body composition, protein, muscle, and nutrient density.

But treatment that is no longer satisfied with telling people to swim upstream while the current remains strong.

The prescription pad must go upstream.

Because people have to eat.

And if we are serious about metabolic health, then what people can afford to eat is not a side conversation.

It is the center of the matter.

In the next chapter, we will extend this upstream thinking beyond food into another powerful determinant of metabolic health: work structure, sleep opportunity, and recovery. But the boldest and clearest upstream intervention in obesity medicine is the one that addresses what patients put in their bodies every single day.

We have financed the rescue.

It is time to help finance the prevention.

Chapter Fourteen: The Respectful Prescription for Work, Recovery, and Human Sustainability

The patient in front of me is not asking for an easier life.

He is asking for support that helps his body sustain the life he has.

He works rotating shifts. Some weeks begin before dawn. Other weeks end after midnight. Meals happen when they can. Sleep happens when it can. The schedule turns before the body has fully caught up. Over time, the waist expands. The blood sugar rises. The snoring worsens. The afternoons get foggier. The hunger gets stranger. He is not sitting in front of me because he does not believe in work. He is sitting in front of me because work, in its current form, is taking a metabolic payment his body is no longer absorbing well.

That distinction matters.

This chapter is not anti-work.

It is not anti-discipline.

It is not anti-productivity.

Work matters. Effort matters. Responsibility matters. A functioning society depends on people showing up, carrying weight, solving problems, and doing difficult things well.

But biology matters too.

And biology keeps its own books.

Earlier in this book, we followed obesity upstream through food engineering, cheap calories, time poverty, short sleep, stress, childhood exposure, and the limits of advice alone. We made room for medication. We made room for surgery. We insisted that body composition matters more than crude scale worship.

We argued, forcefully, that the prescription pad should move upstream toward healthy-food access.

Now we come to a related question, but a more delicate one.

What should a physician say when the structure of work itself has become part of the metabolic story?

That question requires a steadier tone than the food chapter did.

Food access was the bold chapter.

This one has to be the careful chapter.

Because the goal is not to make war on employers. The goal is to tell the truth about recovery.

The body is not only affected by what enters the mouth. It is also affected by when the person sleeps, whether sleep is predictable, whether the day contains real breaks, whether meals are structured or improvised, whether exhaustion has become ordinary, and whether work repeatedly outruns restoration.

The fourth line of the model matters here as much as anywhere in the book.

Calories influence body weight.

Macronutrient balance, especially protein adequacy, influences body composition.

Nutrient density influences health.

And environment determines how hard or easy it is to live out the first three.

That environment includes more than stores and restaurants.

It includes the shift schedule.

It includes the commute.

It includes the break policy.

It includes whether a person can sit down long enough to eat a real meal.

It includes whether bedtime is repeatedly protected or routinely bargained away.

You cannot fully understand obesity without understanding exhaustion.

And you cannot fully understand exhaustion without looking at how work is organized.

Sleep loss changes the next day before breakfast ever arrives.

A short night tends to make hunger louder and fullness less trustworthy. It makes highly rewarding food more persuasive. It makes patience thinner. It makes quick energy look wiser than it really is. A tired brain does not bargain with convenience the way a rested brain does. A tired body also handles blood sugar less gracefully. A tired person is less likely to train, prep food, shop well, or resist the late-afternoon collapse that turns the vending machine or drive-through into a form of relief.

None of that is a character flaw.

It is a physiologic response.

Circadian disruption adds another layer.

Human beings are timed creatures. Hormones, hunger, alertness, glucose handling, temperature regulation, and sleep drive all move through a daily rhythm. When a person repeatedly works at the wrong biological hour, sleeps in fragments, rotates between days and nights, or switches back and forth before the body can adapt, metabolism loses some of its rhythm. Appetite cues get less reliable. Fatigue becomes chronic. Daytime sleep is often shorter and lighter than nighttime sleep. The person may be technically getting “time in bed” without getting the same recovery.

That matters clinically.

The issue is not whether night-shift workers are trying hard enough.

The issue is that circadian misalignment is a real exposure.

And real exposures deserve to be named.

This is especially important because obesity is partly a recovery problem.

An under-recovered body is not starting each day with a fair fight against a hyper-convenient food environment. It is starting from behind. Quick calories feel more justified. Planning feels more expensive. Exercise looks more optional. Protein gets displaced by whatever is easiest. Dinner is asked to repair a day the schedule already destabilized.

That is not laziness.

That is a body making compromised decisions under compromised conditions.

Skipped breaks make the story worse.

Consider the worker whose day leaves no reliable time to eat. The nurse whose patients do not pause for lunch. The driver eating in traffic. The teacher swallowing bites between classes. The warehouse worker grabbing what can be consumed quickly. The physician finishing notes while eating standing up. The office worker who keeps postponing lunch until the hunger is no longer gentle but urgent.

When that pattern repeats, meals stop behaving like structure and start behaving like interruption.

That has consequences.

Protein is often the first casualty of chaotic eating. A deliberately built meal usually contains some thought, some composition, and some protection of fullness. A hurried eating episode often does not. It leans toward what is fast, portable, refined, sweet, salty, and easy to continue. The person may get calories without much satiety. They may get relief without much nourishment. They may get enough energy to keep moving, but not the kind of nutritional support that helps protect lean mass during weight loss or metabolic treatment.

That matters even more in the age of obesity medication.

Earlier in this book, I argued that appetite reduction is not the same thing as treatment completion. When appetite gets quieter, protein must become more intentional, not less. A worker whose appetite is low, schedule is chaotic, and breaks are unreliable can easily drift into a day of under-eating the very foods that would best protect muscle and function. The scale may go down. The body may not be getting stronger. A person can become lighter at work while becoming less physically durable inside that work.

That is not a minor oversight.

It is one of the ways body-composition thinking becomes practical instead of theoretical.

Irregular meals also magnify decision fatigue.

By late afternoon, many workers are not making nutritional decisions from a place of calm judgment. They are making them from accumulated cognitive depletion. The day has already demanded attention, restraint, patience, diplomacy, problem-solving, and task-switching. By evening, convenience has an unfair advantage because the mind is no longer fresh.

This is why simplistic nutrition advice sounds thinner in real life than it does in clinic.

"Plan better" lands differently at 6:30 p.m. after a fully staffed day than it does after a day of understaffing, interruptions, poor sleep, a missed lunch, and a long commute.

That does not mean planning is unnecessary.

It means planning must be built for depletion, not for ideal conditions.

The workplace is therefore not just where people earn a living.

For many adults, it is also one of the places where metabolic stability is either protected or quietly sabotaged.

The question is what medicine should do with that fact.

The first answer is simple.

We should stop pretending it is irrelevant.

If a patient's schedule is materially worsening sleep, appetite regulation, blood sugar control, treatment adherence, or recovery, then the schedule is medically relevant. If repeated missed breaks are contributing to dysregulated eating, poor protein structure, medication timing problems, or worsening metabolic disease, then breaks are medically relevant. If rotating nights are worsening sleep apnea, excessive daytime sleepiness, or a patient's ability to safely manage their chronic disease, then work pattern is medically relevant.

And medically relevant things belong in a physician's field of vision.

That does not mean every physician should become a labor activist. It does not mean every employer conflict belongs inside the exam room. It does not mean medicine should speak carelessly about operations it does not run.

It means physicians should not act as though schedules, fatigue, and recovery are somehow beneath clinical notice when they are clearly shaping health.

The difference between useful advocacy and overreach lies in tone, scope, and discipline.

Useful advocacy is patient-specific.

It is medically grounded.

It is collaborative when possible.

It describes the health issue, the functional strain, and the kind of support that may help.

Overreach sounds different.

It issues broad denunciations.

It moralizes about work itself.

It speaks beyond the physician's expertise.

It tries to manage the employer rather than clarify the medical need.

A physician is not a staffing director.

A physician is not a corporate strategist.

A physician is not a labor attorney.

A physician is a clinician who can say, with authority, that sleep opportunity matters, fatigue matters, predictable recovery matters, protected meal breaks matter, and certain work conditions are materially aggravating a patient's disease.

That is enough.

It is also more powerful than many physicians realize.

There is nothing inherently radical about a health-support letter.

We already write them in many other settings. We recommend work modifications for orthopedic injury. We advise return-to-work limitations after surgery. We document restrictions for pregnancy, chemotherapy, seizure disorders, asthma triggers, or heat exposure. Medicine already knows how to communicate that a body can do some things safely, other things less safely, and some things only if conditions are adjusted.

Obesity-related metabolic strain, sleep disorders, and recovery failure deserve the same seriousness.

The letter does not need to be theatrical.

In fact, it should not be.

The best letters are plain, clinical, and respectful.

"This patient is under active treatment for a medical condition that is worsened by highly variable sleep timing."

"When operationally feasible, a more predictable schedule with fewer rapid rotations would support treatment adherence and recovery."

"This patient would benefit from protected meal breaks sufficient to allow structured nutrition and prescribed medication timing."

"This patient is being treated for significant sleep disruption and daytime fatigue. Repeated quick-return shifts may worsen symptoms and impair recovery."

That is the tone.

Not accusation.

Not ideology.

Not employer denunciation.

Clinical clarity.

The physician should also be disciplined about what not to say.

Do not write as though you are making legal determinations you are not being asked to make.

Do not disclose more diagnosis detail than is necessary.

Do not claim certainty where medicine only supports probability.

Do not prescribe a staffing model for an entire organization based on one patient encounter.

Do not turn a medical letter into a manifesto.

Do not speak in a way that suggests work itself is the enemy.

None of that helps the patient.

And none of it reflects the tone this chapter needs.

The better posture is collaborative seriousness.

A respectful physician can say to an employer, in effect, that this worker is more likely to stay well, function well, and perform more sustainably if sleep timing is less chaotic, recovery more protected, and meal opportunities more reliable.

Most employers can understand that language.

Because the deeper argument is not anti-employer either.

It is pro-durability.

A chronically exhausted workforce is not a high-performing workforce, however admirable its effort may be. Fatigue increases errors. Fatigue increases irritability. Fatigue increases injury risk. Fatigue makes judgment less crisp. Under-recovered workers are more vulnerable to absenteeism, presenteeism, turnover, chronic disease progression, and the long downstream costs that show up later in claims, coverage, disability, and lost continuity.

The precise balance will vary by industry.

But the direction is not mysterious.

Recovery is not the opposite of performance.

Recovery is part of performance.

That sentence deserves to travel.

In some sectors, the most practical reform will not be dramatic. It will be incremental. Better notice of schedules. Fewer abrupt rotations. Fewer "quick return" turnarounds when feasible. Protected break periods that are actually honored. A place to sit down. A real chance to eat before the body hits emergency hunger. Better food defaults in vending machines and cafeterias. Water that is easy to access. Protein-forward options that do not require heroic planning. Less dependence on ultra-processed convenience as the only fuel compatible with a busy shift.

None of that is anti-business.

It is business with a wider definition of operating cost.

Predictability is a metabolic asset.

A predictable sleep window helps the body regulate hormones and appetite more coherently.

A predictable meal window reduces the odds that a worker will ricochet from under-eating to late-day overcorrection.

A predictable break makes it more likely that protein will show up before dinner instead of disappearing from the day.

Predictability lowers friction.

And lower friction is exactly what the fourth line of the model keeps teaching us to care about.

This is why healthier workplace defaults matter more than workplace wellness slogans.

Posters about self-care do not mean very much if the schedule remains chaotic, the breaks remain theoretical, and the only easy food nearby is metabolically weak. Telling employees to be resilient while building days that repeatedly erode resilience is not a serious health strategy.

Defaults matter more than speeches.

If the cafeteria makes the better option easier, some people will take it.

If the vending machine includes protein-rich and less sugar-heavy options, some people will take them.

If the schedule gives enough notice for life to be organized, some families will eat differently.

If the break actually occurs, some workers will stop living on emergency calories.

This is not perfection.

It is friction design.

And friction design is exactly where upstream thinking belongs.

The physician's role in that larger conversation should still remain measured.

We should be able to say that healthy-food access in workplaces matters.

We should be able to say that predictable schedules and protected breaks support treatment adherence and human performance.

We should be able to say that chronic under-recovery is not a minor inconvenience but a disease amplifier.

But we should also avoid pretending that every workplace can instantly remove all strain, or that every job can be reorganized around ideal circadian biology. Some work is inherently around the clock. Hospitals do not close at night. Emergency services do not follow sleep hygiene. Transportation, manufacturing, public safety, and many service sectors require coverage at biologically awkward hours.

That reality should make us pragmatic, not silent.

A pragmatic physician asks, not whether work can be made perfect, but whether it can be made less predictably harmful.

Can the rotations be gentler?

Can the notice be earlier?

Can the break be real?

Can the food be better?

Can the worker with a ciearly documented medical condition be offered more stability when feasible?

Can recovery be treated as part of operational excellence rather than as a private hobby employees are expected to somehow fit in later?

Those are reasonable questions.

They are also respectful ones.

Patients need respectful language here too.

Many readers live under work conditions they cannot easily change. They may be hourly workers, shift workers, caregivers, trainees, business owners, clinicians, or people piecing together several forms of responsibility at once. They do not need this chapter to tell them that the schedule is imperfect. They already know. What they may need is permission to stop interpreting the physiologic consequences as personal weakness.

If that is you, the point is not that your body is failing because you lack discipline.

The point is that the body has real requirements, and those requirements do not disappear just because modern life is busy, respectable, or economically necessary.

Your fatigue is not imaginary.

Your harder hunger after poor sleep is not imaginary.

Your late-day collapse after missed breaks is not imaginary.

The fact that weight management becomes harder when recovery is chronically insufficient is not an excuse.

It is an explanation.

And explanations are useful because they tell us where leverage might exist.

For some patients, that leverage will be medical treatment of sleep apnea.

For some, it will be a better meal structure earlier in the day.

For some, it will be protecting protein more intentionally because appetite is low and work is chaotic.

For some, it will be a carefully written work-support letter.

For some, it will be asking an employer, respectfully, whether a more predictable shift pattern is possible.

For some, it will simply be naming the truth aloud: this body is living in chronic under-recovery, and the treatment plan must be built with that reality in mind.

That last point matters.

A physician should not hand a patient a nutrition fantasy that assumes a calm life the patient does not have. If the patient works nights, the plan has to account for nights. If the patient misses lunch repeatedly, the plan has to defend against missed lunch. If dinner is late and appetite is chaotic, the structure must be designed for the hour that usually breaks. If breaks are unreliable, then portability and protein become even more important. If the schedule rotates, sleep protection becomes part of treatment, not a side note.

A fatigue-tested plan is more respectful than an idealized one.

This is also where physician leadership becomes broader than one letter for one patient.

Healthcare leaders can influence institutional policy. Medical groups can speak to employers with more nuance than the culture often allows. We can advocate for workplace food standards that are not performative. We can support scheduling practices that reduce preventable fatigue without condemning work itself. We can help build a health language that employers can hear without feeling caricatured.

The language should sound like this:

We are not asking you to lower standards.

We are asking you to recognize human operating limits.

We are not asking you to abandon productivity.

We are asking you to protect the conditions that sustain productivity over time.

We are not asking you to infantilize workers.

We are asking you not to design preventable metabolic and cognitive strain into the normal workday when better design is possible.

That is a different moral register from either scolding employers or romanticizing burnout.

It is serious but not shrill.

Collaborative but not timid.

Human but not naïve.

There is still a boundary.

Physicians should be careful not to promise that every schedule change will reverse obesity. Work structure is one upstream driver, not the only one. The food environment still matters. Childhood exposure still matters. Medications still matter. Muscle preservation still matters. Obesity is still multifactorial. This chapter is not claiming that predictability alone cures metabolic disease.

It is making the narrower and more defensible claim.

A physician should be able to advocate for recovery and sustainability without becoming anti-work.

That is the chapter's central sentence.

Work is honorable.

So is sleep.

Discipline matters.

So does restoration.

Productivity matters.

So does durability.

Those are not opposing values unless a system insists on treating them that way.

And systems often do insist on that, which is why this chapter has to end with a larger question than the individual patient, the individual employer, or the individual schedule.

If predictability, recovery, and healthier defaults are good for metabolic health and often good for performance, why are they so often treated as optional?

If employers can see fatigue's effect on errors, turnover, and morale, why does fatigue remain so widely normalized?

If the healthcare system is willing to pay generously for downstream rescue, why does upstream support keep sounding unusual?

Those questions point beyond the clinic.

They point toward incentives.

Toward what gets rewarded.

Toward what the marketplace has been trained to optimize.

Toward the deeper architecture beneath the food supply, the workday, the break room, the schedule, and the daily strain so many bodies are now carrying.

This chapter has argued for a respectful prescription.

Not a war on work.

Not a campaign against employers.

A respectful prescription for more predictability where feasible, more protected recovery, more honest attention to fatigue, and more dignity for the worker whose health is paying the cost.

That prescription is measured by design.

But once we step back far enough, the next question gets sharper.

If the system keeps producing cheap calories, unstable schedules, fragmented sleep, thin margins, and downstream disease, then what exactly is the system being rewarded for producing?

The engine is real.

The question is what the engine has been aimed at.

That is where we turn next.

Chapter Fifteen: The Engine and the Target

The modern food economy did not arise by accident.

It was built.

It was built by intelligent people responding to incentives. It was built by businesses trying to survive and scale. It was built by investors seeking return. It was built by retailers managing margin, shelf life, logistics, and waste. It was built by employers trying to control cost. It was built by insurers trying to manage risk. It was built by policymakers navigating growth, trade, and price stability.

And it worked.

It worked at delivering cheap, durable, convenient calories to millions of people with remarkable efficiency. It worked at making food portable, shelf-stable, profitable, and abundant. It worked at driving down cost per calorie. It worked at filling grocery aisles, vending machines, gas stations, stadiums, airports, and lunchrooms with energy that required very little preparation and almost no planning.

What it did not work at—at least not consistently—was protecting metabolic health.

That is not because markets are evil.

It is because markets are engines.

And engines go where incentives point them.

Blaming "capitalism" for obesity is too crude to be useful. Markets are not moral actors. They are amplifiers. They scale what is rewarded. If the reward structure favors cheap inputs, long shelf life, hyper-palatability, high margin, repeat purchase, and volume sales, then those features will dominate the landscape. If the reward structure favors nutrient density, protein adequacy, satiety, and long-term metabolic resilience, then those features will become more common.

The engine is not the problem.

The target is.

For decades, the target embedded in much of the food economy has been cost per calorie, convenience per minute, and margin per unit. That target makes business sense. It does not automatically make metabolic sense.

The result is what we have been living inside.

An environment where calories are easy to produce, easy to transport, easy to market, easy to consume, and often easier to afford than the foods most likely to support body composition, satiety, and long-term health. An environment where the four-part model repeatedly drifts in the wrong direction at scale:

Calories are easier to exceed.

Protein is easier to neglect.

Nutrient density is easier to displace.

Adherence is harder to sustain.

Then medicine arrives downstream.

We treat high blood sugar. We treat high blood pressure. We treat fatty liver. We treat sleep apnea. We treat joint pain. We prescribe GLP-1-based medications. We perform metabolic surgery. We manage complications with increasing sophistication. We celebrate innovation in rescue while leaving the upstream engine largely untouched.

That imbalance is the moral and strategic failure this book has been tracing from the beginning.

The business of obesity treatment is growing. The business of obesity prevention remains underpowered. That contrast should make us uncomfortable.

Pharmaceutical innovation deserves respect. Bariatric surgery deserves respect. Clinical excellence deserves respect. Patients deserve every effective tool we can offer. But when the incentives in one part of the economy reward calorie-dense, ultra-processed food at scale, and the incentives in another part reward increasingly sophisticated treatment of the resulting disease, we have built a self-reinforcing loop.

The engine produces exposure.

Medicine manages consequence.

The engine keeps running.

This is not an anti-business argument.

It is an incentive argument.

If insurers can reimburse thousands of dollars per month for advanced obesity pharmacotherapy, then the economic system is clearly capable of mobilizing serious capital in response to metabolic disease. If hospitals can finance operating rooms for bariatric surgery, then the system is clearly capable of investing in complex downstream care. If employers can absorb rising healthcare premiums tied in part to obesity-related conditions, then they are already paying for the consequences.

The question is not whether money exists in the system.

The question is what the system chooses to reward.

Right now, the incentives reward low cost per calorie, high shelf stability, hyper-palatability and repeat purchase, portion expansion framed as value, short-term margin over long-term metabolic outcome, and downstream medical billing tied to established disease.

They less consistently reward nutrient density, protein adequacy at scale, portion norms aligned with satiety rather than upsizing, affordable access to minimally processed foods, sleep-protective and recovery-supportive design, and early metabolic stabilization before complications emerge.

The market did not “decide” to harm metabolic health.

It responded rationally to the targets it was given.

This is where economic literacy becomes a professional responsibility for obesity medicine.

If obesity medicine remains purely clinical—if it limits itself to prescriptions, procedures, and counseling inside the exam room—it will remain permanently downstream. It will do honorable work. It will relieve suffering. It will save lives. But it will continue to practice at the bottom of a cliff while the upstream terrain remains tilted toward disease production.

Obesity medicine now has two duties.

The first is to care exceptionally well for the patient in front of us.

The second is to challenge the systems creating the next generation of patients.

Those duties are not in conflict.

They are sequentially incomplete without each other.

The first duty requires precision: body composition, muscle preservation, protein adequacy, sleep assessment, stress awareness, medication when indicated, surgery when appropriate, compassion without stigma, clarity without cruelty.

The second duty requires courage: willingness to say that food design matters, that cheap-calorie economics matter, that school food matters, that healthy-food access should be medically relevant, that incentives can be reoriented, and that physicians are allowed to speak beyond the prescription pad.

Some will hear that and worry that medicine is stepping outside its lane.

It is not.

Medicine has always shaped economic systems. We influence reimbursement structures. We influence benefit design. We influence quality metrics. We influence drug coverage. We influence surgical pathways. We influence what insurers decide to pay for and what employers decide to offer.

The only question is whether we are willing to apply that influence upstream.

Consider a simple contrast.

A physician can prescribe a GLP-1 receptor agonist and unlock insurance coverage worth hundreds or thousands of dollars per month.

That same physician often cannot prescribe subsidized access to vegetables, fruit, high-quality protein, or medically structured grocery benefits with equivalent ease or scale.

If a prescription can unlock coverage for an expensive injectable, a prescription should also be able to unlock access to a diet that does not predictably worsen disease.

That is not anti-market.

It is market rebalancing.

Imagine a food economy where incentives increasingly favored affordable protein-forward staple foods, subsidized produce benefits embedded in healthcare plans, grocery models that reward nutrient density rather than just volume, default portion sizes aligned with satiety instead of upsizing, employer-sponsored food benefits that prioritize metabolic resilience, and institutional food contracts that weight quality and long-term health metrics.

The engine would not disappear.

It would pivot.

The same logistics brilliance that delivers packaged snacks to every corner of the country could deliver protein-rich, nutrient-dense staples at scale. The same marketing sophistication that promotes hyper-palatable convenience foods could elevate healthier defaults. The same capital markets that finance rapid restaurant expansion could finance healthier distribution models when incentives justify it.

Markets follow margin.

If health becomes financially relevant earlier in the chain rather than only at the treatment stage, the engine will respond.

This is not fantasy. It is how systems behave.

We have already seen how rapidly capital flows toward obesity treatment innovation once reimbursement and demand align. Entire industries have reorganized around obesity pharmacotherapy in a matter of years. That speed proves something important: when incentives are clear and strong, change can move quickly.

The next evolution of obesity medicine is not less medicine.

It is wider medicine.

It is a profession that understands biology deeply enough to treat the patient well and understands economics clearly enough to question why the patient needed treatment in the first place.

It is a field that can say, without embarrassment, that:

Protein matters.

Muscle matters.

Nutrient density matters.

Sleep and stress matter.

Cheap calories shape outcomes.

Environment determines adherence at scale.

And that those truths have economic implications.

We do not need to demonize industry. We need to redirect it.

We do not need to dismantle markets. We need to retarget them.

We do not need to vilify profit. We need to align profit with metabolic resilience rather than with passive overconsumption.

This requires a new level of collaboration:

Physicians with business literacy.

Employers who recognize that recovery and metabolic health support long-term performance.

Insurers willing to pay earlier rather than only later.

Food companies that see opportunity in healthier reformulation and better defaults.

Policymakers who understand that healthcare spending already absorbs the cost of upstream design.

The language must remain balanced.

This book has never argued that work is the enemy. Productivity is not the enemy. Markets are not the enemy. Medications are not the enemy. Surgery is not the enemy.

Misaligned incentives are the problem.

If the target rewards disease production, the engine will produce disease.

If the target rewards metabolic resilience, the engine can scale health.

That is the manifesto.

Obesity medicine must stop living only at the bottom of the cliff. It must stop being satisfied with managing the injuries while the terrain above remains unchanged. It must continue to rescue, but it must also insist on redesign.

This is not accusation.

It is responsibility.

The field has matured. It now understands appetite biology more clearly. It has powerful pharmacologic tools. It has surgical expertise. It has a clearer understanding of body composition, muscle preservation, and nutrient density. It has lived through the stigma conversation and emerged with a stronger moral vocabulary.

Now it must become economically fluent.

Because the next decade of obesity medicine will not be defined only by which medication is most effective.

It will be defined by whether we are willing to move the target.

The engine is not the problem.

The target is.

Change the incentives, and the same engine that scaled cheap, convenient calories can scale affordable, accessible, metabolically intelligent food instead.

Care for today's patients with excellence.

Refuse stigma.

Refuse denial.

And then lift the practice of obesity medicine upstream, where the next generation is already being shaped.

That is the work ahead.

Epilogue: Bring the Compass Back to the Middle

At the end of a clinic day, after the exam rooms are quiet and the last patient has gone home, the real size of the problem is easier to feel.

A prescription may have been written. A lab result may have been reviewed. A medication may have been adjusted. A referral may have been placed. A patient may have left with more hope than they arrived with, which is no small thing.

But outside the clinic, the larger system is still running.

The drive-through lanes are still open. The grocery aisles are still full of cheap, durable calories. The school lunch lines will reopen tomorrow. The vending machines will still be waiting. The tired parent will still have to solve dinner after work. The night-shift worker will still sleep against the clock. The child will still learn what food means from the world adults have built around them.

The visit ended.

The exposure did not.

That is the tension at the center of this book.

Obesity medicine has become more powerful. It has better medications, better surgery, better science, and a clearer understanding of appetite, body composition, sleep, stress, and metabolic disease. That progress deserves respect. It is helping real people with real suffering.

But medicine cannot allow its growing power downstream to make it less curious upstream.

A field can become very good at rescue and still be too quiet about why rescue is needed so often.

That is why the compass has to be brought back to the middle.

Not away from patients.

Not away from treatment.

Not away from science.

Back to the place where all of them can be held together honestly.

The country did not suddenly lose willpower. That was the first myth this book had to challenge, because so much harm grows from that single false story. A population-wide pattern deserves a population-level explanation. Millions of people did not simultaneously become less worthy, less disciplined, or less serious about their own lives. The environment changed around them.

Calories became easier to obtain.

Foods became more engineered for speed, reward, and repeat use.

Cheap energy became more available than durable nourishment.

Portions expanded.

Eating opportunities multiplied.

Sleep thinned.

Stress became ordinary.

Time became scarce.

And then a culture surrounded people with these exposures and asked them to interpret the result as private failure.

That story was never honest enough.

It was never compassionate enough.

It was never medically serious enough.

A better story does not erase personal responsibility. It places personal responsibility inside the world where it actually has to operate. People still make choices. Choices still matter. Food matters. Movement matters. Sleep matters. Protein matters. Treatment adherence matters. But choices do not happen in empty space. They happen inside prices, schedules, fatigue, marketing, school food, workplace food, transportation, family stress, sleep debt, and the options close enough to reach when the day has already taken too much.

That is why the fourth line of the model matters so much.

Quantity in calories influences body weight.

Quality of macronutrient balance, especially protein adequacy, influences body composition.

Quality of nutrient density influences health.

Environment determines how hard or easy it is to live out the first three.

The first three lines are biology.

The fourth line is life.

Without that fourth line, nutrition remains clean but incomplete. It tells people what matters without asking whether the world around them makes those truths livable. With the fourth line, the conversation becomes more serious. It becomes less accusatory. It becomes more useful.

It asks not only what a person should do, but what keeps defeating that person's best effort.

It asks not only what the patient knows, but what the patient can actually sustain.

It asks not only how to treat disease after it appears, but how to make disease less likely in the first place.

That is not weakness. It is leadership.

Medicine has done this before. We have learned to see exposures beyond the individual body. We have learned that air quality shapes lung health, that clean water and sanitation prevent infectious disease, that tobacco exposure drives cancer and heart disease, and that road design can prevent or produce traumatic injury. We do not call those insights excuses. We call them public health.

Obesity deserves the same seriousness.

It is a disease of biology, behavior, and environment. It is a disease of appetite and access, fat tissue and food systems, muscle and markets, sleep and schedules, treatment and policy. Any explanation that makes it only one of those things will be too small.

But the wider explanation must remain morally careful.

The purpose of naming obesity as a disease is not to shame people. It is to understand the burden well enough to treat it and prevent it. No one's worth rises or falls with body size, body fat, lab results, or a number on the scale. A person does not become more deserving of respect after weight loss. A child does not become more worthy when they become smaller. An adult living with obesity does not owe the world an apology for being visible.

Dignity is not the prize at the end of treatment.

Dignity is where treatment begins.

At the same time, dignity must not be confused with denial. Excess and dysregulated body fat can burden health. It can worsen blood sugar, liver health, blood pressure, sleep, joint strain, mobility, and daily function. It can make the body harder to live in. It can narrow a person's future options.

Calling that real is not cruelty.

It is care.

The better path is not shame and not silence. It is compassionate clarity. It is the steady medical voice that says: you are not the disease, and the disease still deserves treatment. You are not a failure, and your health still matters. Your worth is settled, and your biology still deserves attention.

That is the balance a humane culture has to recover.

The culture also has to recover a better definition of success.

For too long, weight loss has been treated as if it were the whole prize. But the scale is too crude to carry that much meaning. The goal is not simply to become lighter. The goal is to reduce harmful fat while preserving muscle, protecting function, improving metabolic health, and making the body easier to live in.

A smaller body is not automatically a healthier body.

A healthier body is the goal.

That distinction will matter even more in the years ahead. As medications become more powerful and surgery remains an important option for selected patients, the temptation will be to stare even harder at pounds lost. That would be a mistake. Stronger tools require a stronger definition of success. The question is not only how much weight came off. The question is what kind of tissue was lost, what kind was protected, how the person is functioning, and whether health has truly improved.

Protein matters.

Muscle matters.

Strength matters.

Sleep matters.

Nutrient density matters.

A person should not have to become a smaller, weaker version of themselves in order to be praised by a scale-centered culture.

Obesity medicine can do better than that.

It can be precise enough to protect body composition.

Compassionate enough to reject stigma.

Scientific enough to welcome effective treatment.

And brave enough to admit that treatment is not the same as solution.

That distinction may be the most important one for the profession.

Medications can help. For many patients, they can be life-changing. They can quiet appetite, reduce food preoccupation, improve blood sugar, reduce disease burden, and create room for healthier patterns to take hold.

Surgery can help. For selected patients, bariatric and metabolic surgery can transform health, function, and quality of life. It should not be mocked or dismissed as the easy way out.

These tools matter.

They are not moral failures.

They are not shortcuts around character.

They are treatment for a serious disease.

But rescue is not redesign.

A country cannot fully medicate its way out of a food environment that keeps manufacturing disease. It cannot operate its way out of cheap-calorie economics, chronic under-recovery, childhood exposure, aggressive marketing, and daily defaults that make metabolic health harder than it needs to be.

We need treatment.

And we need more than treatment.

That is the meaning of upstream obesity medicine.

It does not abandon the patient in front of us. It honors that patient more fully by asking why so many patients keep arriving. It does not replace medication or surgery. It places them inside a wider strategy. It does not blame business, work, or markets as if they were inherently wrong. It asks what they are being rewarded to produce.

The engine is not the enemy.

The target is.

Markets can scale disease-promoting defaults when the incentives point that way. They can also scale healthier defaults when incentives are changed. The same brilliance that moves shelf-stable snack foods across a continent can move healthier food if the economic signal becomes strong enough. The same systems that make ultra-processed calories cheap, visible, and convenient can be redirected toward foods that support satiety, protein adequacy, nutrient density, and long-term metabolic health.

That is not fantasy.

It is systems thinking.

The question is whether medicine will help move the target.

If a prescription can unlock coverage for an expensive injectable, a prescription should also be able to unlock access to vegetables, fruit, quality protein, and healthier staple foods for patients whose health depends on them. Food access is not a luxury add-on to obesity medicine. It is one of the most rational upstream interventions available.

People have to eat.

If the food they can afford and access predictably worsens metabolic health, the clinic will keep seeing the result.

That does not mean physicians should control dinner. It means physicians should be able to advocate for medically meaningful nutrition support with the same seriousness we bring to other chronic-disease interventions. It means insurers, health systems, employers, policymakers, and food companies should stop treating healthy food as if it were unrelated to the diseases they are already paying to manage.

The system is already spending money.

The issue is whether it spends only after the damage is done.

Work and recovery deserve a similar, though more measured, place in this reset. Work matters. Productivity matters. Responsibility matters. But sleep, breaks, predictability, and recovery matter too. A tired body does not regulate appetite like a rested one. A worker who never has time to eat a real meal will struggle to protect protein. A parent whose evening has no margin will face a different food environment than a person with time, energy, and a stocked kitchen.

Recovery is not the opposite of performance.

Recovery is part of performance.

That is not anti-work. It is pro-durability. It is a recognition that human beings have operating limits, and that systems ignoring those limits often pay later in fatigue, disease, errors, burnout, and healthcare costs.

This book has not argued for a softer society. It has argued for a wiser one.

A wiser society would not confuse chronic exhaustion with discipline.

It would not confuse cheap calories with true affordability.

It would not confuse body size with moral worth.

It would not confuse scale movement with health.

It would not confuse treatment with solution.

And it would not confuse what is common with what is healthy.

That last confusion may be the most dangerous of all.

A condition can become familiar without becoming benign. A culture can become used to larger portions, shorter sleep, worsening blood sugar, fatty liver, sleep apnea, joint strain, constant snacking, and daily dependence on ultra-processed convenience. The eye adapts. The body does not.

Common is not the same as healthy.

Familiar is not the same as harmless.

If a disease-promoting environment becomes normal, the right response is not to normalize the resulting disease burden. The right response is to redesign the environment.

That redesign will require many kinds of leadership.

Patients and families need a better story than shame.

Clinicians need better tools, better training, and better systems of follow-up.

Healthcare leaders need to pay attention to food access, body composition, sleep, recovery, and prevention.

Insurers need to ask whether paying earlier might be wiser than paying only later.

Employers need practical ways to support healthier food defaults, more predictable recovery where feasible, and human sustainability without abandoning productivity.

Schools need to understand that food exposure, sleep, movement, and habit formation shape the next generation before adult medicine ever sees them.

Food companies need incentives to make metabolically healthier products easier, more appealing, more affordable, and more profitable.

Policymakers need to understand that obesity is not only a private behavior issue. It is a national design issue.

And physicians need to accept that leadership in obesity medicine cannot remain confined to the exam room.

This does not mean medicine should become arrogant. It does not mean physicians have all the answers. We do not. It means we have enough clinical experience to know that the current arrangement is not working well enough. We see the downstream complications. We see the repeated struggle. We see the shame. We see the fatigue. We see the patient who understands the advice but cannot make it survive the world they live in.

That should change us.

It should make us humbler with patients.

It should make us bolder with systems.

The next era of obesity medicine should be defined by that combination: humility downstream, courage upstream.

Humility downstream means meeting the patient with respect. It means asking what they have already tried. It means recognizing the power of appetite, stress, sleep disruption, medications, trauma, genetics, childhood exposure, pain, and environment. It means not assuming that a larger body tells the whole story. It means treating obesity as a disease without treating the person as a problem.

Courage upstream means refusing to stop there. It means asking why healthy food is still harder to access than cheap calories in so many settings. It means asking why the prescription pad is powerful enough to finance rescue but often too weak to finance prevention. It means asking why children are trained so early by a food environment they did not choose. It means asking why the market finds it so easy to scale passive overconsumption and so much harder to scale metabolic resilience.

That work will not be simple.

But difficulty is not the same as impossibility.

Upstream reform is often dismissed as unrealistic because the current system feels so large. But every system that now feels permanent was built by decisions, incentives, habits, and policies that accumulated over time. What was built can be rebuilt. What was rewarded can be rewarded differently. What was normalized can be questioned. What was downstream can be moved upstream.

We do not have to solve everything at once to begin moving in the right direction.

A school can improve its food environment.

A clinic can build a stronger obesity-care pathway.

An insurer can pilot food benefits for high-risk patients.

An employer can protect real breaks and improve cafeteria defaults.

A physician can write differently, speak differently, and lead differently.

A food company can compete on satiety, protein quality, nutrient density, and convenience that does not work against health.

A policymaker can treat food access as healthcare infrastructure.

A family can stop using shame as the language of health.

A patient can stop believing that every past attempt is evidence against their character.

These are not small things.

They are the beginning of a different culture.

That culture will still need treatment. Some people will still need medication. Some will still need surgery. Some will still need intensive clinical support. Some will still struggle despite doing many things right. Obesity will not disappear because the national conversation becomes more intelligent.

But the burden can become less cruel.

The defaults can become less hostile.

The help can arrive earlier.

The language can become cleaner.

The treatment can become more complete.

The prevention can become more serious.

And the patient can stop standing alone at the center of a problem that was never only personal.

That is the hope of this book.

Not a hope built on slogans.

Not a hope that pretends disease is simple.

Not a hope that denies biology, economics, or human frailty.

A steadier hope.

The kind that comes from seeing the map more clearly.

Once we see that obesity is not merely about willpower, we can stop wasting moral energy on blame.

Once we see that weight is not the same as health, we can aim for better outcomes.

Once we see that muscle and function matter, we can protect what should not be sacrificed.

Once we see that sleep, stress, and time poverty shape appetite and adherence, we can build plans that respect the lives people actually live.

Once we see that medications and surgery are tools rather than moral symbols, we can use them wisely.

Once we see that food access is medical, we can begin financing prevention with the seriousness it deserves.

Once we see that markets follow incentives, we can stop cursing the engine and start moving the target.

That is how the compass comes back to the middle.

Not by choosing individual responsibility over systems.

Not by choosing systems over individual responsibility.

Not by choosing treatment over prevention.

Not by choosing prevention over treatment.

Not by choosing compassion over truth.

Not by choosing truth over compassion.

The middle is not weakness. It is balance with a spine.

The country should not confuse common with healthy.

The profession should not confuse treatment with solution.

And patients should not be left carrying responsibility alone for systems that repeatedly work against them.

We do not need less compassion, less science, or less treatment.

We need a wider lens, a stronger spine, and the courage to move the practice of obesity medicine upstream.

Author's Note on Sources and Medical Safety

This book is written for general educational purposes. It is not a clinical practice guideline, a drug label, a nutrition prescription, or individualized medical advice. Obesity, metabolic disease, diabetes, cardiovascular disease, liver disease, sleep apnea, eating disorders, pregnancy, medication use, surgical risk, and other health conditions require individualized evaluation by qualified healthcare professionals.

The central argument of this book is broad: obesity is a complex, chronic, biologically real, environmentally shaped disease; human dignity and medical truth belong together; and treatment should include both compassionate downstream care and serious attention to upstream conditions. The sources below are selected to support that framework. They are intentionally not exhaustive. They are offered as starting points for readers who want to explore the science, guidelines, and public-health thinking behind the book.

Medical Safety Notes

Medical knowledge changes. Medication labels, clinical guidelines, surgical criteria, FDA approvals, insurance coverage, and best-practice recommendations may change after publication. Readers should consult current prescribing information, current clinical guidelines, and their own licensed healthcare professionals before making decisions about medications, surgery, nutrition, physical activity, pregnancy planning, or other health interventions.

The discussion of obesity medications in this book is not an exhaustive medication safety guide. Current FDA-approved labeling and the prescribing clinician's guidance should govern indications, contraindications, pregnancy planning, perioperative management, drug interactions, dosing, monitoring, and serious adverse-effect warnings.

Anti-obesity medications are not appropriate for everyone. Readers should discuss personal and family history, current medications, diabetes therapies, pregnancy or pregnancy plans, breastfeeding, gallbladder disease, pancreatitis history, kidney disease, gastrointestinal symptoms, mood symptoms, prior reactions to medications, and other relevant medical issues with a qualified clinician before starting, stopping, or changing treatment.

Readers using GLP-1 receptor agonists, dual incretin medications, or other obesity medications should seek prompt medical guidance for severe or persistent abdominal pain, repeated vomiting, inability to keep fluids down, signs of dehydration, fainting, jaundice, severe constipation or abdominal distention, symptoms of allergic reaction, significant mood changes, pregnancy, or any other concerning clinical change.

Patients should be cautious about compounded, counterfeit, imported, or casually marketed GLP-1 or related products. Obesity medication should be prescribed within a real clinical relationship and obtained through legitimate, regulated pharmacy channels. Compounded drugs are not the same as FDA-approved drugs, and quality, dosing, sterility, labeling, and safety oversight may differ.

Medication can reduce appetite, but a quieter appetite is not a complete treatment plan. During weight loss—especially when appetite is strongly reduced—protein adequacy, hydration, micronutrient intake, resistance training, strength, function, and medical follow-up still matter. The goal is not simply to become lighter, but to reduce excess fat while preserving health, muscle, and function as much as possible.

Metabolic and bariatric surgery is a serious, evidence-based treatment for selected patients. It should not be dismissed as "the easy way out," and it should not be approached casually. Surgical decisions require individualized evaluation by qualified clinicians and, when appropriate, a multidisciplinary bariatric surgery program. Surgery can be transformative, but it also requires long-term nutrition, supplementation, monitoring, and follow-up.

Nutrition advice should be individualized. Readers with diabetes, kidney disease, heart disease, gastrointestinal disease, food allergies, eating disorder history, pregnancy, frailty, older age, or complex medication regimens should seek professional guidance before making major dietary changes. Readers with a history of eating disorder symptoms should avoid restrictive dieting or weight-loss efforts without appropriate clinical support.

Children and adolescents deserve special care. Childhood obesity should be addressed without shame, humiliation, or cosmetic pressure. Evaluation and treatment should be family-centered, developmentally appropriate, and guided by qualified pediatric clinicians.

Sleep, stress, shift work, time poverty, and recovery are medically relevant, but work and life constraints vary. Any workplace, school, or schedule-related accommodation should be handled through appropriate clinical, occupational, legal, and organizational channels.

Selected Sources and Further Reading

Obesity as a Chronic, Complex Disease

Centers for Disease Control and Prevention. "Consequences of Obesity." CDC, updated 2026.

Centers for Disease Control and Prevention. "Risk Factors for Obesity." CDC, updated 2025.

Wharton S, Lau DCW, Vallis M, et al. "Obesity in Adults: A Clinical Practice Guideline." *Canadian Medical Association Journal*, 2020.

Obesity Canada. *Canadian Adult Obesity Clinical Practice Guidelines*. Obesity Canada, 2020 and subsequent updates.

American Academy of Pediatrics. Hampl SE, Hassink SG, Skinner AC, et al. "Clinical Practice Guideline for the Evaluation and Treatment of Children and Adolescents With Obesity." *Pediatrics*, 2023.

Rubino F, Puhl RM, Cummings DE, et al. "Joint International Consensus Statement for Ending Stigma of Obesity." *Nature Medicine*, 2020.

Food Environment, Diet Quality, and Ultra-Processed Foods

U.S. Department of Agriculture and U.S. Department of Health and Human Services. *Dietary Guidelines for Americans, 2025–2030.* 10th ed. Washington, DC: U.S. Government, 2026.

2025 Dietary Guidelines Advisory Committee. *Scientific Report of the 2025 Dietary Guidelines Advisory Committee.* Submitted to the U.S. Department of Health and Human Services and the U.S. Department of Agriculture, 2024.

Hall KD, Ayuketah A, Brychta R, et al. "Ultra-Processed Diets Cause Excess Calorie Intake and Weight Gain: An Inpatient Randomized Controlled Trial of Ad Libitum Food Intake." *Cell Metabolism*, 2019.

World Health Organization. *Policies to Protect Children From the Harmful Impact of Food Marketing*. WHO guideline, 2023.

American Heart Association. *Food and Beverage Marketing to Children, Adolescents, and Vulnerable Populations*. Policy statement, 2024.

Body Composition, Protein, Muscle, and Physical Activity

Cava E, Yeat NC, Mittendorfer B. "Preserving Healthy Muscle During Weight Loss." *Advances in Nutrition*, 2017.

Leidy HJ, Clifton PM, Astrup A, et al. "The Role of Protein in Weight Loss and Maintenance." *American Journal of Clinical Nutrition*, 2015.

Kim JE, O'Connor LE, Sands LP, Slebodnik MB, Campbell WW. "Effects of Dietary Protein Intake on Body Composition Changes After Weight Loss in Older Adults." *Nutrition Reviews*, 2016.

U.S. Department of Health and Human Services. *Physical Activity Guidelines for Americans*. 2nd edition, 2018.

Piercy KL, Troiano RP, Ballard RM, et al. "The Physical Activity Guidelines for Americans." *JAMA*, 2018.

Sleep, Stress, Shift Work, and Recovery

Watson NF, Badr MS, Belenky G, et al. "Recommended Amount of Sleep for a Healthy Adult: A Joint Consensus Statement of the American Academy of Sleep Medicine and Sleep Research Society." *Journal of Clinical Sleep Medicine*, 2015.

Centers for Disease Control and Prevention. "About Sleep." CDC, updated 2024.

National Institute for Occupational Safety and Health. "Shiftwork, Long Work Hours, and Fatigue." CDC/NIOSH educational materials.

Caruso CC. "Negative Impacts of Shiftwork and Long Work Hours." *Rehabilitation Nursing*, 2014.

Boivin DB, Boudreau P, Kosmadopoulos A. Disturbance of the Circadian System in Shift Work and Its Health Impact. Journal of Biological Rhythms. 2022;37(1):3–28.

Obesity Medications and Medication Safety

U.S. Food and Drug Administration. *Wegovy Prescribing Information*. Current FDA-approved labeling for semaglutide.

U.S. Food and Drug Administration. *Zepbound Prescribing Information*. Current FDA-approved labeling for tirzepatide.

U.S. Food and Drug Administration. "FDA Approves First Treatment to Reduce Risk of Serious Heart Problems Specifically in Adults With Obesity or Overweight." FDA, 2024.

U.S. Food and Drug Administration. "FDA Approves First Medication for Obstructive Sleep Apnea." FDA, 2024.

U.S. Food and Drug Administration. "FDA's Concerns With Unapproved GLP-1 Drugs Used for Weight Loss." FDA, updated 2026.

U.S. Food and Drug Administration. "FDA Alerts Health Care Providers, Compounders and Patients of Dosing Errors Associated With Compounded Injectable Semaglutide Products." FDA, 2024.

Wilding JPH, Batterham RL, Calanna S, et al. "Once-Weekly Semaglutide in Adults With Overweight or Obesity." *New England Journal of Medicine*, 2021.

Jastreboff AM, Aronne LJ, Ahmad NN, et al. "Tirzepatide Once Weekly for the Treatment of Obesity." *New England Journal of Medicine*, 2022.

Pedersen SD, Manjoo P, Dash S, et al. "Pharmacotherapy for Obesity Management in Adults: 2025 Clinical Practice Guideline Update." *Canadian Medical Association Journal*, 2025.

American Diabetes Association Professional Practice Committee for Obesity. Pharmacologic Treatment of Obesity in Adults. Diabetes, Obesity, and Cardiometabolic CARE / BMJ Open Diabetes Research & Care. 2026.

Metabolic and Bariatric Surgery

Eisenberg D, Shikora SA, Aarts E, et al. "2022 American Society for Metabolic and Bariatric Surgery and International Federation for the Surgery of Obesity and Metabolic Disorders: Indications for Metabolic and Bariatric Surgery." *Surgery for Obesity and Related Diseases*, 2022.

American Society for Metabolic and Bariatric Surgery. "After 30 Years—New Guidelines for Weight-Loss Surgery." ASMBS, 2022.

Food Is Medicine, Produce Prescriptions, and Upstream Prevention

Volpp KG, Berkowitz SA, Sharma SV, et al. "Food Is Medicine: A Presidential Advisory From the American Heart Association." *Circulation*, 2023.

Hager K, Cudhea FP, Wong JB, et al. "Impact of Produce Prescriptions on Diet, Food Security, and Cardiometabolic Health Outcomes." *Circulation: Cardiovascular Quality and Outcomes*, 2023.

U.S. Department of Health and Human Services, Office of Disease Prevention and Health Promotion. *U.S. Department of Health and Human Services / ODPHP. Food Is Medicine Landscape Summary. 2024.*

U.S. Department of Health and Human Services. *Food Is Medicine Research Needs*. 2024.

The Aspen Institute Food & Society Program. *Food Is Medicine Research Action Plan*. 2024.

Closing Note to Readers

This book does not ask readers to choose between personal responsibility and systems thinking, or between treatment and prevention. It argues that both are necessary. Individuals deserve practical, compassionate, evidence-based care. They also deserve environments that make health easier to sustain. The sources above are offered in that spirit: not as a complete scientific archive, but as a transparent trail into the medical, nutritional, behavioral, surgical, and public-health evidence that informs the book.

www.ingramcontent.com/pod-product-compliance
Lightning Source LLC
LaVergne TN
LVHW100307210926
848480LV00003B/1043